U0397029

Operating Specifications for Distinctive External Therapies of Zhuang Medicine

壮医特色外治法操作规范

（中英文版）

主 编 李 铭 郑光珊 翟 阳

Editor-in-Chief Li Ming Zheng Guangshan Zhai Yang

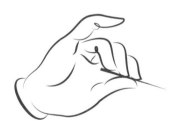

广西科学技术出版社

Guangxi Science & Technology Publishing House

图书在版编目（CIP）数据

壮医特色外治法操作规范：汉文、英文 / 李铭，郑光珊，翟阳
主编.—南宁：广西科学技术出版社，2023.5
ISBN 978-7-5551-1923-4

Ⅰ.①壮… Ⅱ.①李… ②郑… ③翟… Ⅲ.①壮医—中医外科—汉、英
Ⅳ.①R291.8

中国版本图书馆CIP数据核字（2023）第034842号

ZHUANGYI TESE WAIZHIFA CAOZUO GUIFAN

壮医特色外治法操作规范（中英文版）

主编 李 铭 郑光珊 翟 阳

责任编辑：黎志海 吴桐林		装帧设计：梁 良
责任校对：吴书丽		责任印制：韦文印

出 版 人：卢培钊	出版发行：广西科学技术出版社
社 址：广西南宁市东葛路 66 号	邮政编码：530023
网 址：http://www.gxkjs.com	

经 销：全国各地新华书店
印 刷：广西昭泰子隆彩印有限责任公司
开 本：787 mm×1092 mm 1/16

字 数：249 千字	印 张：14.75
版 次：2023 年 5 月第 1 版	印 次：2023 年 5 月第 1 次印刷

书 号：ISBN 978-7-5551-1923-4
定 价：128.00 元

编委会名单

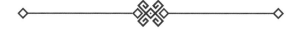

顾　问：黄瑾明　黄汉儒

主　审：岳桂华　黄国东

主　编：李　铭　郑光珊　翟　阳

副主编：潘明甫　贺诗寓　罗远带

编　委（按姓氏笔画排列）：

马　威　王秋风　韦进新　韦国彪　卢　敏

朱红梅　农田泉　刘　莉　许夏懿　苏本兰

巫文岗　杨　鹏　杨秀静　杨雪桦　李凤珍

吴　丹　何　亮　邹　敏　张　莹　张安东

张洪瑞　陈　莹　陈超群　林　琴　罗盼盼

周　红　周明钊　施明华　莫宇凤　唐　静

唐菀玲　黄小薇　黄世威　黄敏婷　梅小平

龚珊鸿　蒋咏玲　蒋桂江　覃丽萍　温　勇

谭海丽　潘惠萍

翻　译：李举先 @ 语言桥

资助项目：1. 2022 年中医药国际交流与合作项目

　　　　　2. 广西科技基地和人才专项（桂科 AD18281094）

List of Editorial Board Members

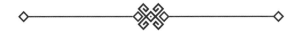

Funded projects：1. 2022 TCM International Exchange and Cooperation Project
2. Guangxi Science and Technology Base and Talents Project
（Guike AD18281094）

目　录
Contents

第一章　壮医药线点灸疗法
Chapter 1　Zhuang Medicine Medicated Thread Moxibustion

第二章　壮医神龙灸疗法
Chapter 2　Zhuang Medicine Shenlong Moxibustion

第三章　壮医针刺疗法
Chapter 3　Zhuang Medicine Acupuncture Therapy

第四章　壮医莲花针拔罐逐瘀疗法
Chapter 4　Zhuang Medicine Stasis-Removing Therapy with Lotus-Needling and Cupping

第五章　壮医刮痧疗法
Chapter 5　Zhuang Medicine Skin Scraping Therapy

第六章 壮医烫熨疗法
Chapter 6 Zhuang Medicine Ironing Therapy

第七章　壮医药物竹罐疗法
Chapter 7　Zhuang Medicine Bamboo Cupping Therapy

第八章　壮医刺血疗法
Chapter 8　Zhuang Medicine Pricking Blood Therapy

第九章　壮医火攻疗法
Chapter 9　Zhuang Medicine Fire Therapy

第十章　壮医香囊佩药疗法
Chapter 10　Zhuang Medicine Medicated Sachet Therapy

第十一章　壮医经筋推拿疗法
Chapter 11　Zhuang Medicine Meridian Sinew（Jing Jin）Massage Therapy

第十二章　壮医火针疗法
Chapter 12　Zhuang Medicine Fire-Needle Therapy

第十三章　壮医针挑疗法
Chapter 13　Zhuang Medicine Needle-Pricking Therapy

第十四章　壮医包药疗法
Chapter 14　Zhuang Medicinal Materials Bag Therapy

第十五章　壮医全身药浴疗法
Chapter 15　Zhuang Medicine Whole Body Medicated Bath Therapy

第十六章　壮医敷贴疗法
Chapter 16　Zhuang Medicine Application Therapy

第十七章　壮医滚蛋疗法
Chapter 17　Zhuang Medicine Egg-Rolling Therapy

第十八章　壮医水蛭疗法
Chapter 18　Zhuang Medicine Leech Therapy

第一章　壮医药线点灸疗法
Chapter 1　Zhuang Medicine Medicated Thread Moxibustion

壮医药线点灸疗法是用壮药泡制的苎麻线点燃后，直接灼灸患者体表的一定穴位或部位，以治疗疾病的一种方法。

Zhuang medicine medicated thread moxibustion refers to a therapeutic method of pressing the burning ramie thread which is soaked in Zhuang medicinal liquor on some acupoints or parts by a certain skill.

一、主要功效
Ⅰ　Main effects

祛风、湿、疹、瘴、寒、痰等毒，通调三道两路，调节气血平衡，补虚强体等。

To dispel wind，dampness，pathogen，miasma，cold and phlegm. To regulate three passages and two pathways（note：three passages including grain passage，qi passage and water passage are related to the generation，storage，transformation，and excretion of nutrition in the body；two pathways include dragon route referring to the route for the blood circulation and fire route referring to the route for the sensory transmission），regulate the balance between qi and blood，restore vital energy，improve physical health，etc.

二、适应证
Ⅱ　Indications

内科、外科、妇科、儿科、五官科、皮肤科等常见病、多发病均可使用本疗法治疗，常见适应证有唪呗啷（带状疱疹、带状疱疹后遗神经痛）、能啥累（瘙痒、湿疹）、发得（发热）、得凉（感冒、上呼吸道感染）、喯佛（包块肿块）、唅尹（疼痛）、发旺（痹病）、麻抹（麻木）、巧尹（头痛）等。

This therapy can be used to treat common diseases and frequently-occurring diseases of internal medicine，surgery，gynecology，pediatrics，ENT，dermatology，etc. Its common indications include Benbeilang（shingles，postherpetic neuralgia），Nenghanlei（pruritus，eczema），Fade（fever），Deliang（cold，upper respiratory tract infection），Benfo（lump），Benyin（pain），Fawang（arthralgia disease），Mamo（numbness），Qiaoyin（headache），etc.

三、禁忌证
Ⅲ　Contraindications

（1）严重心脑血管疾病患者、血糖控制不佳者、精神病患者、身体极度消瘦虚弱患者等禁用。

（1）It is prohibited for patients who have severe cardiovascular and cerebrovascular diseases，poor glycemic control，psychosis，or an extremely weak constitution.

（2）眼球、男性外生殖器龟头部和女性小阴唇部禁灸。

（2）It is prohibited on the eyeball，the glans or labia minora.

（3）黑痣慎用。

（3）It should be used cautiously on the melanotic nevus.

（4）过度疲劳、过度饥饿、过度饱或精神高度紧张的患者禁用。

（4）It is prohibited for patients who suffer from excessive fatigue，excessive hunger，overeating or high mental stress.

（5）孕妇禁用。

（5）It is prohibited for pregnant women.

四、操作前准备
Ⅳ　Preparations before operation

（1）环境要求。治疗室内清洁，安静，光线明亮，温度适宜，避免患者吹风受凉。

（1）Environmental requirements. The treatment room should be clean，quiet，well-lit. Besides，keep the treatment room at an ideal temperature to prevent the patient from catching a cold.

（2）用物准备。药线（苎麻线，大号直径约 1 mm、中号直径约 0.7 mm、小号直径约 0.25 mm，图 1-1）、生理盐水、消毒棉签、一次性无菌手套、酒精灯、打火机、镊子、剪刀（图 1-2）。

（2）Materials preparation. Medicated thread（ramie thread，the diameters of its large size，medium size，and small size are about 1 mm，0.7 mm，and 0.25 mm respectively）（Fig. 1-1）. Physiological saline，sterile cotton swabs，disposable sterile gloves，an alcohol lamp，a lighter，a pair of tweezers，a pair of scissors（Fig. 1-2）.

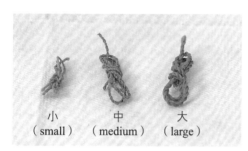

图 1-1　药线分类

Fig. 1-1　Classification of medicated thread

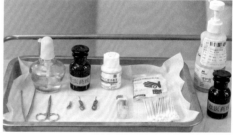

图 1-2　其他用物准备

Fig. 1-2　Preparation of other materials

（3）操作前护理。核对患者信息及治疗方案等，向患者说明治疗的意义和注意事项，取得患者同意；对患者进行精神安慰与鼓励，消除患者的紧张、恐惧情绪，使患者能积极主动配合操作。

（3）Nursing care before operation. The nurse should check the patient's information and treatment plan and explain the significance and notices of the treatment to obtain the patient's consent. Besides，the nurse should encourage the patient to overcome his/her nervousness and fear and enable the patient to cooperate with the doctor for a better operation.

五、操作步骤

V　Operation procedures

（1）体位选择。根据患者病情确定体位，常取坐位、俯卧位、仰卧位、侧卧位等，以患者舒适及便于施术者操作为宜，避免用强迫体位。

（1）Posture selection. Based on the state of the illness, the posture is determined. Sitting position, prone position, dorsal position or lateral recumbent position is often selected to provide convenience for the patient and the doctor. The compulsive position should be avoided.

（2）定穴。根据病证选取对应的治疗部位。取穴原则："寒手热背肿在梅，痿肌痛沿麻络央，唯有痒疾抓长子，各疾施灸不离乡。"

（2）Acupoints location. According to the disease patterns, the corresponding treatment area is selected. Principles of acupoint selection, "Acupoints on the hand should be selected to treat cold diseases. Acupoints on the back should be selected to treat fever. Plum blossom acupoints（a group of acupoints are selected to form the shape of a plum blossom according to the shape and size of lump and Plum blossom acupoints are applied to treat the diseases of internal medicine and lump）should be selected to treat swelling. Sunflower acupoints（a group of acupoints are selected to form the shape of a sunflower according to the shape and size of skin lesion and Sunflower acupoints are applied to treat skin diseases）should be selected to treat dermatomycosis. Acupoints on the part of muscle atrophy should be selected to treat muscle atrophy. Acupoints on the pain part should be selected to treat pain. Acupoints on numb part should be selected to treat numbness. Acupoints on itchy part should be selected firstly to treat itching".

（3）洗手，戴医用外科口罩、医用帽子，非常规手法施术者须戴一次性无菌手套。

（3）The doctor should wash hands, wear a surgical mask and a medical cap. Besides, the doctor who performs unconventional manipulation needs to wear disposable sterile gloves.

（4）清洁。用生理盐水清洁要施灸的皮肤。

（4）Cleaning. Clean treatment areas with physiological saline.

（5）施术流程。

（5）Operation procedures.

①取线。用镊子从药液中取出药线。

① Thread taking. The doctor takes the thread out of medicinal liquor with a pair of tweezers.

②整线。将松散的药线搓紧、拉直（图1-3）。

② Thread twisting. The doctor tightens and straightens up the loose thread（Fig. 1-3）.

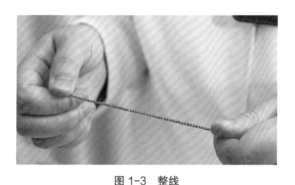

图 1-3　整线

Fig. 1-3　Thread twisting

③持线。

③ Thread holding.

常规手法：右手食指和拇指指尖相对，持药线的一端，露出线头1～2 cm；药线另一端卷入掌心（图1-4）。

Conventional manipulation：The doctor holds one end of the medicinal thread with the index finger and thumb tip of one hand. Moreover，the length of the exposed end of the medicinal thread should be 1 ～ 2 cm and the other end of the medicinal thread should be held in the palm of the hand（Fig. 1-4）.

非常规手法：用像针刺持针一样的方法持药线的一端，露出线头2～5 cm；药线另一端卷入掌心（图1-5）。

Unconventional manipulation：The doctor holds one end of the medicinal thread just as the needle holding of acupuncture. Moreover，the length of the exposed end of the medicinal thread should be 2 ～ 5 cm and the other end of the medicinal thread should be held in the palm of the hand（Fig. 1-5）.

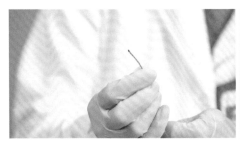 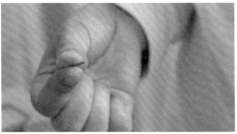

图 1-4　常规手法
Fig. 1-4　Conventional manipulation

图 1-5　非常规手法
Fig. 1-5　Unconventional manipulation

④点火。将露出的线端在酒精灯火上点燃（图1-6），使线头有圆珠状炭火星，称珠火（图 1-7）。

④ Thread igniting. The doctor ignites the exposed end of the medicinal thread on an alcohol lamp（Fig. 1-6）to make the flame turn to be a cylinder-like charcoal fire（Fig. 1-7）.

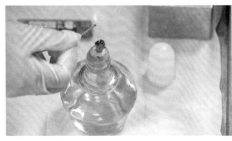 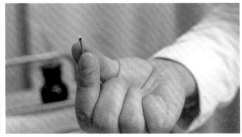

图 1-6　点火
Fig. 1-6　Thread igniting

图 1-7　线头有圆珠状炭火星
Fig. 1-7　Making the flame turn to be a cylinder-like charcoal fire

⑤施灸。

⑤ Thread moxibustion.

常规手法：将药线的炭火星线端对准穴位或治疗部位，顺应手腕和拇指的屈曲动作，拇指指腹迅速地将珠火的线头直接点按在穴位或治疗部位上（图1-8）。一按珠火灭即起为 1 壮。

Conventional manipulation：The doctor holds the medicinal thread with thumb and index finger of one hand，and then presses the burning end directly on the acupoints or treatment areas with the flexion movement of both wrist and thumb （Fig. 1-8）. One burning of medicinal thread in this therapy is called one cone.

非常规手法：将线端珠火直接刺灸在穴位或治疗部位上，无拇指点按动作（图 1-9）。珠火灭即起为 1 壮。

Unconventional manipulation：The doctor directly stings acupoints or treatment areas with cylinder-like charcoal fire without the thumb pressing（Fig. 1-9）. One burning of medicinal thread in this therapy is called one cone.

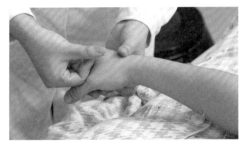 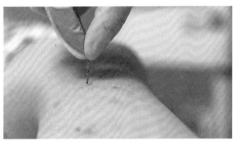

图 1-8　常规手法施灸　　　　　　　图 1-9　非常规手法施灸
Fig. 1-8　Conventional manipulation　　　Fig. 1-9　Unconventional manipulation

（6）整理患者衣物及操作物品。

（6）The doctor tidies up the patient's clothing and used materials.

（7）交代患者治疗后注意事项等。

（7）The doctor informs the patient of precautions after treatment.

（8）洗手并记录治疗情况。

（8）The doctor washes hands to make a record about treatment.

六、疗程
Ⅵ　Course of treatment

一般每穴（莲花、葵花等除外）点灸 1～3 壮。急性病疗程较短，一般每天灸 1 次，5～7 天为 1 个疗程。慢性病则疗程较长，可每隔 2～3 天灸 1 次，

15 ～ 20 天为 1 个疗程。

In general, one to three burning of medicinal thread are applied to acupoints（except Lotus acupoints, Sunflower acupoints, etc.）. The course of treatment for acute diseases is short（once a day and 5 to 7 days as a course of treatment）. While the course of treatment for chronic diseases is long（once every three to four days and 15 to 20 days as a course of treatment）.

七、注意事项

Ⅶ　Notes

（1）患者过度疲劳、过度饥饿、过度饱或精神高度紧张时不能操作。暴露治疗部位时，应注意保护患者隐私及保暖。

（1）It is prohibited for patients who suffer from excessive fatigue, excessive hunger, overeating or high mental stress. When the treatment part is exposed, the doctor should protect the patient's privacy and keep patient warm.

（2）一般情况下应用常规手法进行点灸治疗，但点灸口腔部位，或局部有破溃、渗液处，或传染性皮肤病患者，施术者必须戴一次性无菌手套，使用非常规操作手法，不可直接接触患处，避免交叉感染。

（2）In general case, conventional manipulation is used in this therapy. However, when the doctor performs this therapy in patient's oral cavity, or the patient has ulcer and exudation areas on skin, or infectious skin disease, the doctor must wear disposable sterile gloves and use unconventional manipulation to perform this therapy. The doctor should not touch the affected area directly to avoid cross infection.

（3）注意手法轻重。施灸时，珠火接触穴位或治疗部位时间短，点灸壮数少者为轻手法，适用于面部穴位及未成年患者。珠火接触穴位或治疗部位时间较长，点灸壮数较多者为重手法，适用于癣类疾病、足底穴位或急救时。珠火接触穴位的时间及点灸壮数介于轻手法和重手法之间者为中手法，适用于一般疾病。

（3）Pay attention to the manipulation. The mild manipulation should be applied to the situation that the cylinder-like charcoal fire is pressed on the acupoints or treatment areas for a short time and the number of burning of medicinal thread in moxibustion is small. It is suitable for facial acupoints. Besides, the doctor also can perform this manipulation to minor patients. The intense manipulation is applied to the situation that the cylinder-like charcoal fire is pressed on the acupoints or treatment areas for a long time and the number of burning of medicinal thread in moxibustion is large. It is suitable for ringworm diseases, acupoints on the sole or first aid. The moderate manipulation is applied to the situation that the time of cylinder-like charcoal fire being pressed on the acupoints is between the time of the above-mentioned two manipulations, and the times of burning of medicinal thread in moxibustion is between the times of the above-mentioned two manipulations. It is suitable for common diseases.

（4）点火时，如有火苗应轻柔抖灭，不可用嘴巴吹灭。

（4）If there is a flame, it should be gently shaken until it disappears, and it should not be blown out by mouth.

（5）药线点燃以后，只有珠火适用，以线端火星最旺时为点灸良机，以在点灸部位留下药线白色炭灰为效果最佳。

（5）After the medicinal thread is ignited, only the cylinder-like charcoal fire is applicable. When the medicinal thread has the brightest spark, it is the best time to do this therapy and the best effect can be achieved when white medicinal thread ash is left on the treated areas.

（6）点灸外眼区及面部靠近眼睛的穴位时，嘱患者闭目，避免火花飘入眼内引起烧伤。

（6）When applying this therapy to acupoints near the patient's eyes or on external parts of the eye, the doctor should tell the patient to close his/her eyes to prevent sparks from burning the eyes.

（7）施灸过程中随时观察患者局部皮肤及病情，随时询问患者对点灸的耐受程度。

（7）During this process, the doctor should observe the patient's local skin and condition as well as ask the patient's tolerance to this therapy at any time.

（8）操作后交代患者，局部会出现浅表的灼伤痕迹，停止点灸 1～2 周后可自行消失。若施灸部位有瘙痒或轻度灼伤，属正常治疗反应。避免用手抓破，以免引起感染；若不小心抓破，注意保持清洁或用碘伏消毒。

（8）After the operation, the doctor should explain to the patient that superficial burn marks will be left on the skin, and it will disappear on its own within one to two weeks after stopping this therapy. It is a normal reaction that there is itching or mild burns on treated areas after treatment. The patient should not scratch the itchy or burnt area to avoid infection; in case the itchy or burnt area is broken by scratching, keep the area clean or disinfect it with iodophor.

（9）治疗后在饮食上应注意忌口（如皮肤病，在点灸治疗期间忌食牛肉、公鸡肉、鲤鱼等发物），以清淡饮食为主。

（9）Diet should be paid attention to after the treatment. The patient who has skin disease should avoid eating beef, rooster meat, carp and other stimulating food, and have a bland diet during treatment.

八、意外情况及处理
Ⅷ　Accidents and handling methods

（1）晕灸。如患者在点灸过程中出现气短、面色苍白、出冷汗等晕灸现象，应立即停止操作，让患者头低位平卧并服少量糖水。

（1）Fainting. If the patient develops shortness of breath, pale complexion and cold sweat during this therapy, this operation should be stopped immediately, and help the patient lie flat with head-down tilt and let him/her drink a small amount of sugar water.

（2）烫伤、起水疱。如烫伤，用生理盐水清洁创面并浸润无菌纱布湿敷创面，直至疼痛明显减轻或消失后，外涂烧伤膏。如起小水疱，皮肤可自行吸收，保持局部干燥及水疱皮肤的完整性即可。

（2）Burns and blisters. For burns, the surface of the wound should be cleaned with physiological saline and compressed by wet sterile gauzes until the pain is greatly relieved or disappears, and then applied burn ointment. For small blisters, the skin will absorb the blisters fluid if the skin over the blisters is not open and kept dry.

【附注】
【Notes】

壮医药线制备
The Preparation of Medicinal Thread

（1）材料制作。将苎麻浸水湿润，搓成大、中、小 3 种规格的苎麻线，大号直径约 1 mm、中号直径约 0.7 mm、小号直径约 0.25 mm。将搓好的苎麻线泡在火灰水中 10 天进行脱脂处理，也可以用纯碱代替火灰。如果急用，可用 5% 纯碱水煮苎麻线 1 小时即可达到脱脂的目的。取出用清水洗净晒干。

（1）Materials preparation. The ramie threads are soaked in water and twisted into large，medium and small sizes. The diameters of its large size，medium size，and small size are about 1 mm，0.7 mm，and 0.25 mm，respectively. Then，the twisted ramie threads will be soaked in water with plant ashes for 10 days for degreasing. The sodium carbonate（soda）can be used to replace plant ashes. For urgent use，the doctor can boil the twisted ramie thread in 5% soda water for one hour. Then，the twisted ramie thread should be taken out，cleaned with the fresh water and dried.

（2）药液制作（参考）。先取当归藤 50 g、肿节风 50 g、飞龙掌血 50 g、过江龙 50 g 等壮药，加入 45 度米酒共浸泡于瓶内，再将苎麻线浸入以上药液中，密封浸泡。

（2）Preparation of medicinal solution（for reference）. Firstly，Dangguiteng（*Embelia parviflora* Wall.）50 g，Zhongjiefeng（Herba Sarcandrae）50 g，Feilongzhangxue（Radix Toddaliae Asiaticae）50 g，Guojianglong（Complanate Clubmoss Herb）50 g，other Zhuang medical materials and rice wine（45% vol）are put in a bottle. Secondly，the twisted ramie threads are soaked in this solution and then the bottle is sealed.

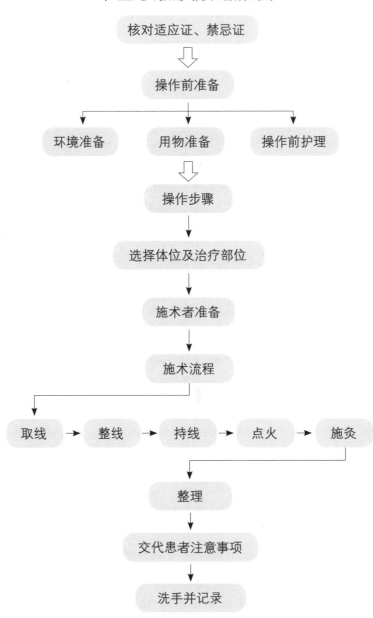

壮医药线点灸疗法流程图

核对适应证、禁忌证

操作前准备

环境准备　用物准备　操作前护理

操作步骤

选择体位及治疗部位

施术者准备

施术流程

取线 → 整线 → 持线 → 点火 → 施灸

整理

交代患者注意事项

洗手并记录

The Flow Chart about Zhuang Medicine Medicated Thread Moxibustion

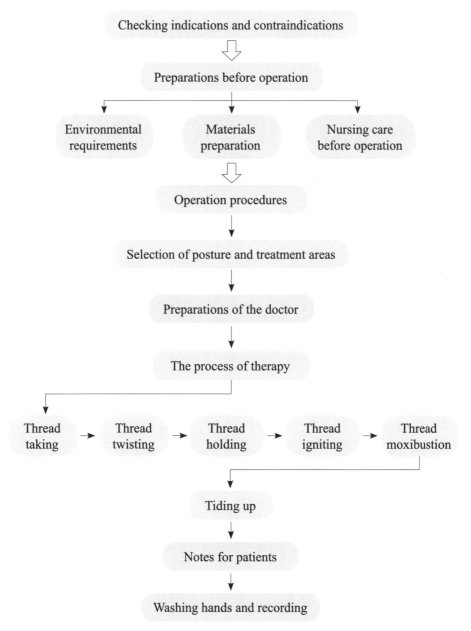

第二章　壮医神龙灸疗法
Chapter 2　Zhuang Medicine Shenlong Moxibustion

壮医神龙灸疗法是通过在人体背部或胸腹部施灸，用姜渣及艾绒的辛散温通之力治疗疾病的一种方法。

Zhuang medicine Shenlong moxibustion refers to a therapeutic method of applying moxibustion on patient's back，chest or abdomen with ginger residue and moxa which are warming the body to dissipate cold to treat diseases.

一、主要功效
Ⅰ　Main effects

祛风、湿、寒、痰、瘀等毒，止痛，补虚，通调三道两路，调节气血平衡。

To dispel wind，dampness，cold，phlegm and blood stasis. To relieve pain，restore vital energy，regulate three passages and two pathways and the balance between qi and blood.

二、适应证
Ⅱ　Indications

内科、外科、妇科、五官科、皮肤科等常见病、多发病均可使用本疗法治疗，常见适应证有楞涩（鼻炎）、得凉（感冒、上呼吸道感染）、奔唉（咳嗽）、奔墨（哮喘）、年闹诺（失眠）、麻邦（中风）、令扎（强直性脊柱炎）、发旺（痹病）、核嘎尹（腰腿痛）、活邀尹（颈椎病）、旁巴尹（肩周炎）、麻抹（麻木）、甬裆呷（半身不遂）、兰奔（头晕）、嗙呗啷（带状疱疹、带状疱疹后遗神经痛）、腊胴尹（腹痛）、京尹（痛经）、约京乱（月经不调）、卟很裆（不孕）、巧尹（头痛）、勒爷屙细（小儿泄泻）、嘞内嘘内（虚劳）等。

This therapy can be used to treat the common diseases and frequently-occurring diseases of internal medicine，surgery，gynecology，ENT，dermatology，etc. Its common indications include Lengse（rhinitis），Deliang（cold，upper respiratory tract infection），Ben'ai（cough），Benmo（asthma），Niannaonuo（insomnia），Mabang（stroke），Lingzha（ankylosing spondylitis），Fawang（arthralgia disease），Hegayin（lumbocrural pain），Huoyaoyin（cervical spondylosis），Pangbayin（scapulohumeral periarthritis），Mamo（numbness），Bengdangxia（hemiplegia），Lanben（dizziness），Benbeilang（shingles，postherpetic neuralgia），Ladongyin（abdominal pain），Jingyin（dysmenorrhea），Yuejingluan(irregular menstruation)，Buhendang(infertility)，Qiaoyin(headache)，Leye'exi（infantile diarrhea），Leineixunei（ deficiency ），etc.

三、禁忌证
Ⅲ Contraindications

（1）辨证为阳证患者禁用。

（1）It is prohibited for patients with Yang syndrome.

（2）发热（体温≥ 37.3 ℃）、脉搏≥ 90 次 / 分患者禁用。

（2）It is prohibited for patients with fever（body temperature ≥ 37.3 ℃）or pulse rate ≥ 90 beats/min.

（3）有开放性创口或感染性病灶者禁用。

（3） It is prohibited for patients with open wounds or infectious lesions.

（4）过度疲劳、过度饥饿、过度饱或精神高度紧张的患者禁用。

（4）It is prohibited for patients who suffer from excessive fatigue，excessive hunger，overeating or high mental stress.

（5）严重心脑血管疾病患者、血糖控制不佳者、精神病患者、身体极度消瘦虚弱患者等禁用。

（5）It is prohibited for patients who have severe cardiovascular and cerebrovascular diseases，poor glycemic control，psychosis，or an extremely weak constitution.

（6）孕妇禁用。

（6）It is prohibited for pregnant women.

四、操作前准备

Ⅳ　Preparations before operation

（1）环境要求。治疗室内通风，清洁，安静，光线明亮，温度适宜，避免患者吹风受凉。

（1）Environmental requirements. The treatment room should be clean, quiet, well-lit. Besides, keep the treatment room at an ideal temperature to prevent the patient from catching a cold.

（2）用物准备。姜渣（图2-1）、艾绒（图2-2）、桑皮纸、灸器（图2-3），95%酒精、95%酒精棉球、喷壶、酒精灯、打火机、止血钳、治疗单、毛巾、无菌纱布、压板、一次性无菌手套（图2-4）。

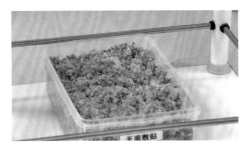

图 2-1　姜渣

Fig. 2-1　Ginger residue

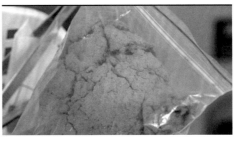

图 2-2　艾绒

Fig. 2-2　Moxa

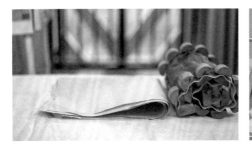

图 2-3　桑皮纸及灸器

Fig. 2-3　Mulberry paper and moxibustion device

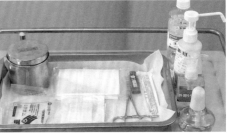

图 2-4　其他物品

Fig. 2-4　Other materials

（2）Materials preparation. Ginger residue（Fig. 2-1）, moxa（Fig. 2-2）, mulberry paper, moxibustion device（Fig. 2-3）, 95% alcohol, 95% alcohol cotton balls, a watering can, an alcohol lamp, a lighter, a hemostat, the treatment sheet, towels, sterile gauzes, a spatula, disposable sterile gloves（Fig. 2-4）.

（3）操作前护理。核对患者信息及治疗方案等，向患者说明治疗的意义和注意事项，取得患者同意；对患者进行精神安慰与鼓励，消除患者的紧张、恐惧情绪，使患者能积极主动配合操作。

（3）Nursing care before operation. The nurse should check the patient's information and treatment plan and explain the significance and notices of the treatment to obtain the patient's consent. Besides, the nurse should encourage the patient to overcome his/her nervousness and fear and enable the patient to cooperate with the doctor for a better operation.

五、操作步骤
V　Operation procedures

（1）体位选择。根据患者病情确定体位，常取俯卧位、仰卧位等，以患者舒适及便于施术者操作为宜，避免用强迫体位。

（1）Posture selection. Based on the state of the illness, the corresponding posture is selected. Prone position or dorsal position is often selected to provide convenience for the patient and the doctor. The compulsive position should be avoided.

（2）部位选择。取背廊穴（包括龙脊、夹脊）或脐线。

（2）Position selection. Dorsovisceral points（including Longji, Jiaji）or umbilical line are selected.

（3）洗手，戴医用外科口罩、医用帽子及一次性无菌手套。

（3）Wash hands, wear a surgical mask, a medical cap and disposable sterile gloves.

（4）施术流程。

（4）Operation procedures.

①放灸器。再次评估施灸部位皮肤情况，将桑皮纸铺在患者施灸部位（图

2-5），灸器放在桑皮纸上（图 2-6）。

① Putting the moxibustion device. The skin condition of treatment areas is evaluated again and the mulberry paper is spread on treatment areas（Fig. 2-5），then，the moxibustion device is put on the mulberry paper（Fig. 2-6）.

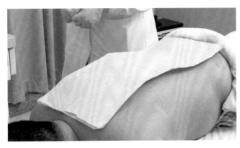

图 2-5　铺桑皮纸

Fig. 2-5　Putting the mulberry paper

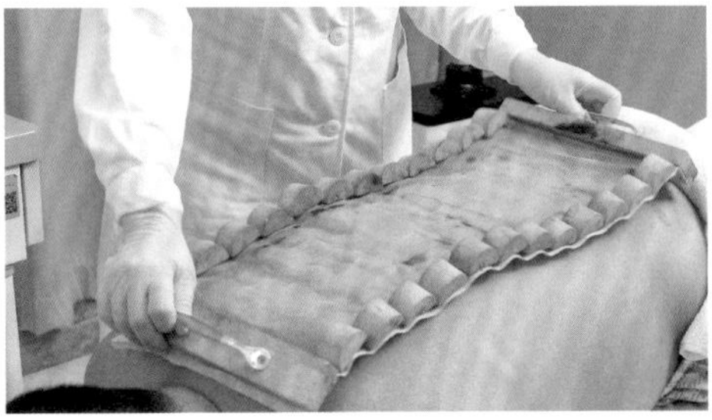

图 2-6　放灸器

Fig. 2-6　Putting the moxibustion device

②铺姜渣。将姜渣放在手中压紧后放入灸器，铺满，厚 2～3 cm（图 2-7）。

② Spreading the ginger residue. The doctor puts the ginger residue in his/her hands and presses it tightly. Then，the doctor spreads the ginger residue on the moxibustion device with the thickness of 2 to 3 cm（Fig. 2-7）.

③铺艾绒。将厚 1～2 cm 的艾绒放在手中压成扁平状后铺在姜渣上（图 2-8）。

③ Spreading the moxa. The doctor puts the moxa with a thickness of 1 to 2 cm in the hand，and then presses it into a flat shape and spreads it on the ginger residue （Fig. 2-8）.

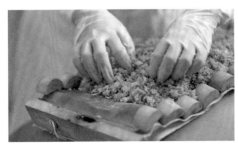

图 2-7　铺姜渣

Fig. 2-7　Spreading the ginger residue

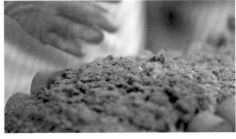

图 2-8　铺艾绒

Fig. 2-8　Spreading the moxa

④燃艾绒。用喷壶将 95% 酒精均匀喷洒在艾绒上（图 2-9），点燃艾绒使药力迅速升温通达龙脊，此为 1 壮。待第 1 壮艾绒燃烧至大部分焦黑后，另取艾绒放在手中压成扁平状后铺撒在第 1 壮艾绒上，取 95% 酒精棉球点火沿龙脊自上而下点燃艾绒（图 2-10）。每次可灸 2 ～ 5 壮，以患者自觉施灸部位温煦发热为宜。

④ Burning the moxa. Put the 95% alcohol into a watering can and spray it on the moxa evenly（Fig. 2-9）, and ignite the moxa to enhance the drug efficacy quickly on the Longji acupoint. This is called one burning of moxa in moxibustion. After most moxa are charred, the doctor takes some moxa again in his/her hand and presses it into a flat shape, spreads it on the charred moxa, ignite a 95% alcohol cotton ball to ignite the moxa along Longji acupoint from up to down（Fig. 2-10）. 2 to 5 burning of moxa in moxibustion can be selected each time to make the patient feel warm on his/her treated areas.

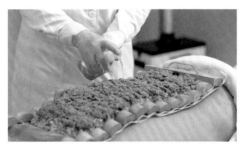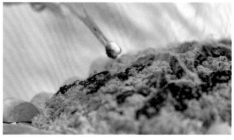

图 2-9　喷酒精　　　　　　　　　　　图 2-10　点艾绒
Fig. 2-9　Spraying alcohol　　　　　　　Fig. 2-10　Igniting the moxa

⑤观察。随时询问患者耐热感受。如患者诉温度过高，可将压板插入灸器下平行滑动以隔热及散热（图 2-11）；或短暂轻抬灸器，观察患者皮肤情况。

⑤ Observation. Ask the patient's tolerance to heat at any time. If the patient complains that the temperature is too high, put a spatula under the moxibustion device and slide it for heat insulation and heat dissipation（Fig. 2-11）or lift the moxibustion device lightly to observe the patient's skin condition.

⑥灸毕。确认艾绒燃烧完毕，撤除灸器（图 2-12）并抬至治疗车下层，将桑皮纸放入医疗垃圾桶。检查患者皮肤，用无菌纱布轻拭施灸部位的水迹后，

立即给患者覆盖被子予以保暖。

⑥ Finishing the moxibustion. After confirming that the moxa has been burned out，remove the moxibustion device（Fig. 2-12），and put it to the lower layer of the treatment cart，put the mulberry paper into the medical trash can. Then，check the patient's skin，wipe the water on treated areas with sterile gauzes，and immediately cover the patient with a quilt to keep him/her warm.

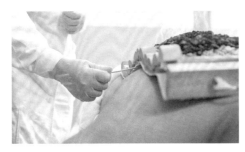

图 2-11　隔热散热 | 图 2-12　撤除灸器
Fig. 2-11　Heat insulation and heat dissipation | Fig. 2-12　Removing moxibustion device

（5）整理患者衣物及操作物品。

（5）The doctor tidies up the patient's clothing and used materials.

（6）交代患者治疗后注意事项等。

（6）The doctor informs the patient of precautions after treatment.

（7）洗手并记录治疗情况。

（7）The doctor washes hands and makes a record about treatment.

六、疗程
Ⅵ　Course of treatment

3～7天灸1次，3～5次为1个疗程。

Once every 3 to 7 days，3 to 5 times for a course of treatment.

七、注意事项
VII　Notes

（1）患者过度疲劳、过度饥饿、过度饱或精神高度紧张时不能操作。暴露治疗部位时，应注意保护患者隐私及保暖。

（1）It is prohibited for patients who suffer from excessive fatigue，excessive hunger，overeating or high mental stress. When the treatment part is exposed，the doctor should protect the patient's privacy and keep the patient warm.

（2）灸后注意观察皮肤情况，施灸后皮肤出现微红灼热或轻微瘙痒，属正常现象，无须处理。

（2）Pay attention to the skin condition after moxibustion. It is normal that the skin is with reddish color，a burning sensation or slight itching feeling after moxibustion.

（3）治疗后4～6小时内不宜洗澡，注意保暖，避免吹风着凉。

（3）It is not advisable to take a bath within 4 to 6 hours after treatment. Keep warm and avoid catching a cold.

（4）治疗当天避免过量运动，忌食寒凉、热性及酸辣刺激、肥甘厚味、鱼腥等食物。

（4）Avoid excessive exercise on the treatment day and foods that are cold，spicy，sour，greasy and fishy should be avoided.

八、意外情况及处理
VIII　Accidents and handling methods

（1）晕灸。如患者在点灸过程中出现气短、面色苍白、出冷汗等晕灸现象，应立即停止操作，让患者头低位平卧，亦可加服少量糖水；若患者严重至昏迷不醒，应立即行急救处理。

（1）Fainting. If the patient develops shortness of breath，pale complexion and cold sweat during the moxibustion，this operation should be stopped immediately，and help the patient lie flat with head-down tilt and let him/her drink a small amount of sugar water. If the patient is unconscious，an emergency treatment should be performed immediately.

（2）烫伤、起水疱。如烫伤，用生理盐水清洁创面并浸润无菌纱布湿敷创面直至疼痛明显减轻或消失，外涂烧伤膏。如起小水疱，皮肤可自行吸收，保持局部干燥及水疱皮肤的完整性即可；如水疱较大，可用无菌针头将水疱戳破，放出疱内渗液，每日用碘伏消毒，外涂烧伤膏，保持局部干燥及清洁，预防感染。

（2）Burns and blisters. For burns，the surface of the wound should be cleaned with physiological saline and compressed by wet sterile gauzes until the pain is greatly relieved or disappears，and then applied burn ointment. For small blisters，the skin will absorb the blisters fluid if the skin over the blisters is not open and kept dry. For large blisters，a sterile needle can be used to puncture them to release the fluid. Then disinfect it with iodophor，apply burn ointment to it，and keep the skin dry and clean every day to prevent infection.

【附注】
【Notes】

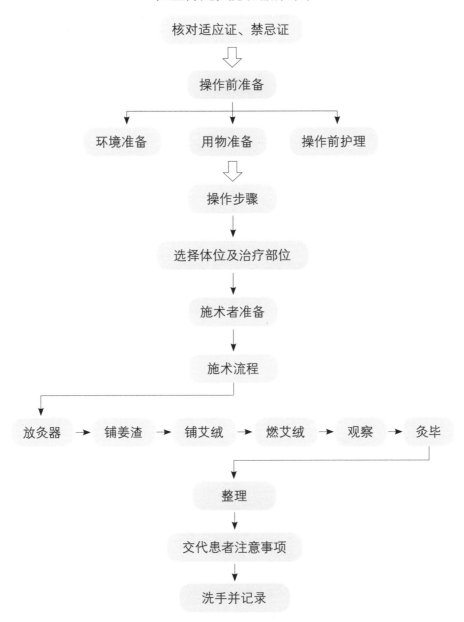

壮医神龙灸疗法流程图

The Flow Chart about Zhuang Medicine Shenlong Moxibustion

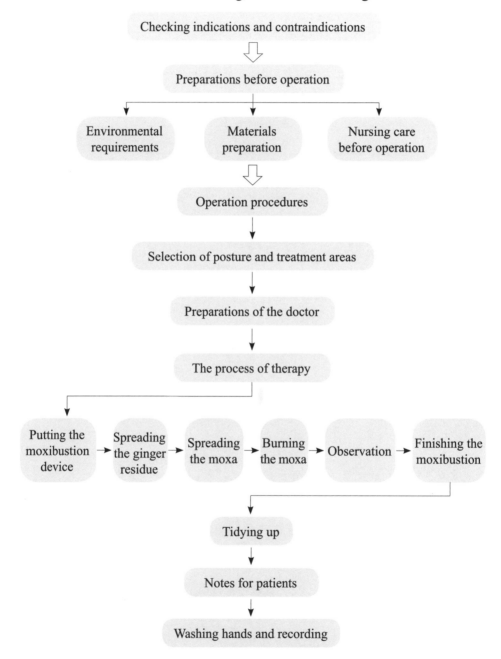

第三章 壮医针刺疗法
Chapter 3　Zhuang Medicine Acupuncture Therapy

　　壮医针刺疗法是以壮医理论和壮医临床思维方法为指导，在人体一定的穴位或部位上运用针具刺入，以疏通三道两路、调节气血平衡、恢复脏腑功能而治疗疾病的一种方法。

　　Zhuang medicine acupuncture therapy is based on the theory and clinical practices of Zhuang medicine. It uses needles to act on acupoints to regulate three passages and two pathways, the balance between qi and blood and restore the function of viscera.

一、主要功效
Ⅰ　Main effects

　　祛风、湿、痧、瘴、寒、热、痰等毒，散结，通痹，消肿，活血，通络，止痛，通调三道两路，调节气血平衡，促进人体自愈。

　　To dispel wind, dampness, pathogen, miasma, cold, fever and phlegm. To eliminate stagnation, arthralgia spasm and swelling. To promote blood circulation, dredge collaterals and relieve pain. To regulate three passages and two pathways, the balance between qi and blood, restore vital energy and improve physical health.

二、适应证
Ⅱ　Indications

　　内科、外科、妇产科、男科、儿科、皮肤科、五官科等临床常见病、多发病及疑难杂症均可使用本疗法治疗。常见适应证有发旺（痹病）、年闹诺（失眠）、核嘎尹（腰腿痛）、活邀尹（颈椎病）、旁巴尹（肩周炎）、麻邦（中风）、甬裆呷（半身不遂）、麻抹（麻木）、兰奔（头晕）、巧尹（头痛）、唪呗啷（带状疱疹、带状疱疹后遗神经痛）、腊胴尹（腹痛）、京尹（痛经）、约京乱（月经不调）、卟很裆（不孕）、楞涩（鼻炎）、奔鹿（呕吐）、能啥累（瘙痒、湿疹）等。

This therapy can be used to treat the common diseases, frequently-occurring diseases and difficult miscellaneous diseases of internal medicine, surgery, gynecology, andrology, pediatrics, dermatology, ENT, etc. Its common indications include Fawang（arthralgia disease）, Niannaonuo（insomnia）, Hegayin（lumbocrural pain）, Huoyaoyin（cervical spondylosis）, Pangbayin（scapulohumeral periarthritis）, Mabang（stroke）, Bengdangxia（hemiplegia）, Mamo（numbness）, Lanben（dizziness）, Qiaoyin（headache）, Benbeilang（shingles, postherpetic neuralgia）, Ladongyin（abdominal pain）, Jingyin（dysmenorrhea）, Yuejingluan（irregular menstruation）, Buhendang（infertility）, Lengse（rhinitis）, Benlu（vomiting）, Nenghanlei（pruritus, eczema）, etc.

三、禁忌证
Ⅲ Contraindications

（1）孕妇慎用，孕期亦禁刺手十甲穴等一些具有通龙路、火路作用的穴位。

（1）It should be used cautiously for pregnant women. Besides, it is prohibited for pregnant women to perform acupuncture on some acupoints which can regulate dragon route and fire route such as Shijia acupoint.

（2）小儿囟门未闭合时，头顶部的穴位不宜针刺。

（2）When the fontanel is not closed, the acupoints on the vertex of infants are not suitable for acupuncture.

（3）患者皮肤有感染、溃疡、疤痕或肿瘤的部位及凝血功能障碍者禁用。

（3）It is prohibited for patients whose skin have infection, ulcers, scars or tumors. Besides, it is also prohibited for patients with coagulation disorders.

（4）过度疲劳、过度饥饿、过度饱或精神高度紧张的患者禁用。

（4）It is prohibited for patients who suffer from excessive fatigue，excessive hunger，overeating or high mental stress.

四、操作前准备
Ⅳ　Preparations before operation

（1）环境要求。治疗室内清洁，安静，光线明亮，温度适宜，避免患者吹风受凉。

（1）Environmental requirements. The treatment room should be clean，quiet，well-lit. Besides，keep the treatment room at an ideal temperature to prevent the patient from catching a cold.

（2）用物准备。内盛各种型号的一次性毫针（管针）的治疗盘、复合碘皮肤消毒液、棉签、弯盘、大浴巾、脉枕、一次性利器盒（图 3-1）。

（2）Materials preparation. A medical tray containing various types of disposable filiform needles（pipe needles），compound iodine skin disinfectant，sterile cotton swabs，a curved tray，large bath towels，a wrist cushion for the doctor to feel patient's pulse，a disposable sharps box（Fig. 3-1）.

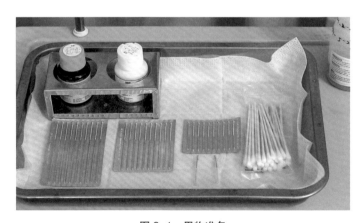

图 3-1　用物准备

Fig. 3-1　Materials preparation

注意，应根据患者的性别、年龄、胖瘦、体质、病情、病灶穴位来选取长短、粗细适宜的针具。《灵枢·官针》指出："九针之宜，各有所为，长短大小，各有所施也。"男性及体壮、形胖且病位较深者，可选取稍粗、稍长的毫针，如直径超过 0.3 mm、长 2～3 寸的针具；女性及体弱、形瘦而病位较浅者，则应选用较短、较细的针具，如直径 0.2～0.25 mm、长 1～2 寸的针具。

The lengths and diameters of the needles should be selected based on the patient's gender，age，stature，physique，disease condition，lesions and the acupoints. *Spiritual Pivot · Acupuncture*（*Lingshu · Guanzhen*）has pointed out，"The key points of acupuncture lie in the proper selection of needles. Needles in different sizes and lengths have various usages." Choose the slightly large and long needles that are more than 0.3 mm in diameter and 2 to 3 cun（1 cun ≈ 3.3 cm）in length for men and strong and obese patients with deep lesion. Choose the slightly short and small needles that are 0.2 to 0.25 mm in diameter and 1 to 2 cun in length for women and weak and thin patients with shallow lesion.

（3）操作前护理。核对患者信息及治疗方案等，向患者说明治疗的意义和注意事项，取得患者同意；对患者进行精神安慰与鼓励，消除患者的紧张、恐惧情绪，使患者能积极主动配合操作。

（3）Nursing care before operation. The nurse should check the patient's information and treatment plan and explain the significance and notices of the treatment to obtain the patient's consent. Besides，the nurse should encourage the patient to overcome his/her nervousness and fear and enable the patient to cooperate with the doctor for a better operation.

五、操作步骤
V　Operation procedures

（1）体位选择。根据患者病情确定体位，常取坐位、俯卧位、仰卧位、侧卧位等，以患者舒适及便于施术者操作为宜，避免用强迫体位。

（1）Posture selection. Based on the state of the illness，the posture is selected. Sitting position，prone position，dorsal position or lateral recumbent position is often selected to provide convenience for the patient and the doctor. The compulsive position should be avoided.

（2）部位选择。经过壮医望、闻、按、探、诊五诊合参后根据患者病情轻重缓急和症状确定施针穴位。

（2）Position selection. The doctor identifies patient's disease condition and symptoms by combining inspection，auscultation and olfaction，hand-feeling diagnosis，medium-based diagnosis and inquiry in Zhuang medicine，and then selects acupoints.

（3）洗手，戴医用外科口罩、医用帽子。

（3）The doctor should wash hands，wear a surgical mask and a medical cap.

（4）消毒。

（4）Disinfection.

①部位消毒。用复合碘皮肤消毒液消毒皮肤（由内向外环消毒，直径大于5 cm）。

① Skin disinfection. The skin is disinfected by the compound iodine skin disinfectant（the direction of disinfection is from inside to outside，the diameter of disinfection area is more than 5 cm）.

②施术者消毒。施针前先用酒精棉球或棉签消毒持针的手指（图 3-2）。

② Self-disinfection. The doctor should use an alcohol cotton ball or cotton swab to disinfect the fingers that will hold the needles before acupuncture（Fig. 3-2）.

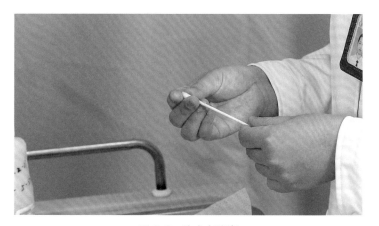

图 3-2　施术者消毒

Fig. 3-2　Self-disinfection

（5）施术流程。

（5）Operation procedures.

壮医针刺疗法根据患者的体质、症状和体征分为补法、泻法和平补平泻法。此外，还有壮医特定穴针刺疗法——脐环穴针刺疗法。

Zhuang medicine acupuncture therapy method is divided into three types: reinforcing method, reducing method, neutral supplementation and draining method. The doctor adopts these methods to treat diseases according to the patient's constitution, symptoms and signs. In addition, there is an acupuncture method for specific acupoints in Zhuang medicine—acupuncture at the umbilical ring acupoints.

①补法。

① Reinforcing method.

进针。根据腧穴深浅和患者体形选择合适的毫针。嘱患者做腹式呼吸运动。执针，将毫针对准穴位，并趁患者吐气时将针刺入穴位至适宜深度（图3-3）。

Needle inserting. The right filiform needle is selected based on the depth of the acupoints and the patient's habitus. The patient is instructed to do abdominal respiratory movement. The doctor holds the needle, finds the right acupoint, and inserts the needle into the acupoint in appropriate depth when the patient is exhaling（Fig. 3-3）.

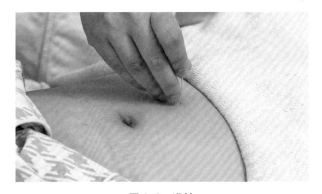

图 3-3　进针

Fig. 3-3　Needle inserting

具体的进针深度除由穴位部位特点决定外，临床上还需灵活掌握。如形体瘦弱者宜浅刺，形体肥胖者、青壮年、身体强壮者宜深刺；年老者、体弱者、小儿宜浅刺；阳证、初病者宜浅刺，阴证、久病者宜深刺；头面部、胸背部及肌肉薄处宜浅刺，四肢、臀部、腹部及肌肉丰厚处宜深刺；手指足趾、掌跖部宜浅刺，肘臂、腿膝处宜深刺；等等。针刺的角度和深度有关，一般来说，深刺多用直刺，浅刺多用斜刺和平刺。对颈项后正中、大动脉附近、眼区、胸背部的穴位，尤其要掌握斜刺深度、方向和角度，以免造成患者损伤。注：泻法、平补平泻法进针深度原则同补法。

The specific depth of the needle inserting is determined by the characteristics of the selected acupoint, and it is flexible in clinical practice. Shallow needling is suitable for thin patients. Deep needling is suitable for obese, young or strong patients. Shallow needling is suitable for the elderly and the patients with weak constitution as well as children. Shallow needling is suitable for patients with Yang syndrome and at the onset of the disease. Deep needling is suitable for patients with Yin syndrome or long-term illness. Shallow needling is suitable for head, face, chest, back and thin muscles. Deep needling is suitable for limbs, buttock, abdomen and thick muscles. Shallow needling is suitable for fingers, toes and palmoplantar. Deep needling is suitable for elbows, arms and knees. The angle of acupuncture is related to the depth. In general, deep needling can be carried out with perpendicular insertion while shallow needling can be performed with oblique insertion and horizontal insertion. Pay attention to the depth, direction and angle of oblique needling for the acupoints on the posterior median of the neck, eye area, chest and back, near the large artery so as to avoid damage. Note: The principles about the depth of needle inserting of reducing method and neutral supplementation and draining method are the same as those of reinforcing method.

留针候气。进针完毕后，可留针候气（图3-4），待"气至"后再行运针吐纳补泻治疗手法。壮医以三道两路为传导和调节系统，判定"气至"，不以酸、麻、胀为标准，而是以针体自行摆动、有下坠针感、针口皮肤高起或陷落（或红晕）为标准，只要出现其中一项即可视为"气至"。一般情况下，留针20～40分钟以候气。

Prolonged needling for acu-esthesia. The doctor can perform prolonged needling for acu-esthesia after the needle inserting (Fig. 3-4). Then, the doctor performs respiratory reinforcing and reducing method with the needles after qi arrives. Zhuang medicine takes three passages and two pathways as the transmission and regulation systems to determine whether qi arrives or not. Signs of the qi arrival is not that patients feel the soreness, numbness and distension but the doctor feels a dragging and/or tensense sensation, or there is skin bulge, skin depression or flare around the needle. In general, the time of prolonged needling for acu-esthesia is 20 to 40 minutes.

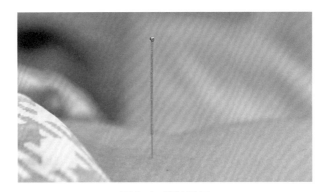

图 3-4 留针候气
Fig. 3-4　Prolonged needling for acu-esthesia

运针吐纳施补。按三气同步理论，施术者将针提起少许，迅速插下，连续9次（通常取奇数，由施术者灵活掌握），然后嘱患者做腹式吐纳运动，连续3次（通常取奇数，由施术者灵活掌握）。上述过程即为给该穴位施补1次。每位患者需要在哪些穴位进行施补，每个穴位施补几次，视病情而定。若行提插时患者诉疼痛，立即改轻微捻转（图3-5）替代提插。施补的目的是调节三气同步，针感并非首要，必须尽量避免让患者感到疼痛。

The doctor performs respiratory reinforcing method by twirling the needle. According to the theory of three-qi harmony, the doctor lifts the needle, then quickly inserts it. This process needs to be performed 9 times in a row（odd number, it is flexibly mastered by the doctor）, and then the doctor asks the patient to do abdominal respiratory movement, another 3 times in a row（odd number, it is flexibly mastered by the doctor）is performed. The above process is one reinforcing method performent for the acupoint. The selection of acupoints and the frequency of each acupoint for reinforcing method by needling depend on the patient's disease condition. When the patient complains of pain while the doctor is lifting and thrusting the needle, the doctor should slightly twirl the acupuncture needle immediately（Fig. 3-5）. The purpose of performing the reinforcing method is to regulate three-qi harmony. The needling sensation is not the most important and the doctor should try to keep patients from feeling pain.

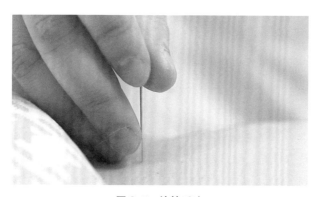

图 3-5　捻转手法
Fig. 3-5　Twirling the needle

出针。嘱患者做腹式吐纳运动，趁患者纳气时将针缓慢拔出。出针后立即用消毒棉签按压针孔，并轻轻揉按几次，防止气血外泄及出血。

Withdrawing the needle. The patient is instructed to perform abdominal respiratory movement, and then the needle is withdrawn. The pinhole should be pressed with a sterile cotton swab immediately after withdrawing the needle. Then, press the pinhole gently several times to prevent bleeding and the leakage of qi.

②泻法。

② Reducing method.

进针。根据腧穴深浅和患者体形选择合适的毫针。嘱患者做腹式吐纳运动。执针，将毫针对准穴位，并趁患者吐气时将针刺入穴位至适宜深度。具体进针深度原则同补法。

Needle inserting. The right filiform needle is selected based on the depth of the selected acupoints and the patient's habitus. The patient is instructed to do abdominal respiratory movement. The doctor holds the needle, finds the right acupoint, and inserts the needle into the acupoint in appropriate depth when the patient is exhaling. The principle about the depth of needle inserting of reducing method is the same as that of reinforcing method.

留针候气。进针完毕后，待"气至"再行运针吐纳补泻治疗手法。一般情况，留针时间为 20 分钟，还可以依据患者病情需要，延长留针至 30 ～ 50 分钟。

Prolonged needling for acu-esthesia. The doctor performs prolonged needling for acu-esthesia after the needle inserting. Then，the doctor performs respiratory reinforcing and reducing method with the needle after the qi arrival. In general，the time of prolonged needling for acu-esthesia is 20 minutes. Besides，the time of prolonged needling for acu-esthesia can be extended to 30 to 50 minutes according to the patient's disease condition.

运针吐纳施泻。按三气同步理论，施术者将针提起少许后迅速插下（图 3-6），连续 6 次（通常取偶数，由施术者灵活掌握），然后嘱患者做腹式吐纳运动，连续 4 次（通常取偶数，由施术者灵活掌握），上述过程即为给该穴位施泻 1 次。每位患者需要在哪些穴位进行施泻，每个穴位施泻几次，视病情而定。若行提插时患者诉疼痛，立即改轻微捻转替代提插。施泻的目的是调节三气同步，针感并非首要，必须尽量避免让患者感到疼痛。

The patient is performed respiratory reducing method. According to the theory of three-qi harmony，the doctor lifts the needle，then quickly inserts it（Fig. 3-6）. This process needs to be performed 6 times in a row（even number，it is flexibly mastered by the doctor），and then the doctor asks the patient to do abdominal respiratory movement，another 4 times in a row（even number，it is flexibly mastered by the doctor）is performed. The above process is one reducing method performent for the acupoint. The selection of acupoints and the frequency of each acupoint for reducing method by needling depend on the patient's disease condition. When the patient complains of pain while the doctor is lifting and thrusting the needle，the doctor should slightly twirl the acupuncture needle immediately. The purpose of performing the reducing method is to regulate three-qi harmony. The needling sensation is not the most important and the doctor should try to keep patients from feeling pain.

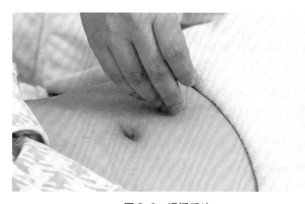

图 3-6 提插手法

Fig. 3-6 Lifting and thrusting the needle

出针。嘱患者做腹式吐纳运动，趁患者吐气时将针缓慢拔出。出针后立即用消毒棉签按压针孔，并轻轻揉按几次，防止气血外泄及出血。

Withdrawing the needle. The patient is instructed to perform abdominal respiratory movement，and then the needle is withdrawn. The pinhole should be pressed with a sterile cotton swab immediately after withdrawing needle. Then，press the pinhole gently several times to prevent bleeding and the leakage of qi.

③平补平泻法。

③ Neutral supplementation and draining method.

进针。根据腧穴深浅和患者体形选择合适的毫针。嘱患者做腹式呼吸运动。执针，将毫针对准穴位，并趁患者吐气时将针刺入穴位至适宜深度。具体进针深度原则同补法。

Needle inserting. The right filiform needle is selected based on the depth of the selected acupoints and the patient's habitus. The patient is instructed to do abdominal respiratory movement. The doctor holds the needle，finds the right acupoint，and inserts the needle into the acupoint in appropriate depth when the patient is exhaling. The principle about the depth of needle inserting of neutral supplementation and draining method is the same as that of reinforcing method.

留针候气。进针完毕后，一般情况下，留针时间为 20 分钟，也可以依据患者病情需要，延长留针至 30 ~ 50 分钟，中间无须提插或捻转。

Prolonged needling for acu-esthesia. In general，the time of prolonged needling for acu-esthesia is 20 minutes. Besides，the time of prolonged needling for acu-esthesia can be extended to 30 to 50 minutes according to the patient's disease condition. There is no need to lift，thrust and twirl the acupuncture needle.

出针。嘱患者做腹式吐纳运动，趁患者吐气或纳气时将针缓慢拔出（图3-7）。出针后立即用消毒棉签按压针孔，并轻轻揉按几次，防止气血外泄及出血。

Withdrawing the needle. The patient is instructed to perform abdominal respiratory movement，and then the needle is withdrawn（Fig. 3-7）. The pinhole should be pressed with a sterile cotton swab immediately after the needle is withdrawn. Then，press the pinhole gently several times to prevent bleeding and the leakage of qi.

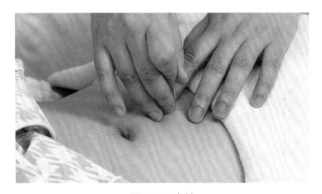

图 3-7　出针
Fig. 3-7　Withdrawing the needle

④壮医特定穴针刺疗法——脐环穴针刺疗法。

④ Acupuncture method for specific acupoints in Zhuang medicine—acupuncture at the umbilical ring acupoints.

选针。使用 0.25 mm×25 mm 的一次性无菌毫针（1 寸管针）。

Needle selection. Disposable sterile filiform needles（1 cun pipe needles）of 0.25 mm×25 mm are selected.

取穴。在脐窝的外侧缘旁开 0.2 寸做一圆环，环线上均为穴位。将脐内环看成一个钟表，以脐中央（神阙）为钟表的中心，根据脏腑归属分别在 12 点时位、1 点 30 分时位、3 点时位、4 点 30 分时位、6 点时位、7 点 30 分时位、9 点时位、10 点 30 分时位 8 个点上取穴（图 3-8）。

Acupoints selection. A ring with 0.2 cun away from the lateral margin of umbilicus is made. Related acupoints are on it. The umbilical ring is regarded as a clock and the umbilical center（Shenque acupoint）is regarded as the center of the clock. Acupoints are selected according to the positions of the hour hand（12 o'clock, half past 1, 3 o'clock, half past 4, 6 o'clock, half past 7, 9 o'clock and half past 10）which correspond to zang-fu's normal position in the body（Fig. 3-8）.

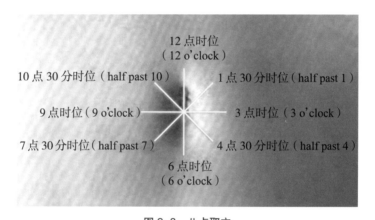

图 3-8　八点取穴

Fig. 3-8　Acupoints selection at 8 points

进针。进针前，嘱患者先做腹式吐纳运动，调整好呼吸，平稳情绪，消除紧张感，然后采用管针无痛进针（图 3-9）。以脐为中心，向外呈 10°角放射状平刺，进针深度约为 0.8 寸（图 3-10）。

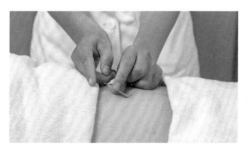

图 3-9　管针进针

Fig. 3-9　Needle inserting of the pipe needle

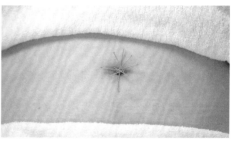

图 3-10　脐环针展示

Fig. 3-10　Display of needles on the umbilical ring acupoints

Needle inserting. The patient is instructed to perform abdominal respiratory movement before the needle inserting to adjust breathing，stabilize mood and overcome nervousness. Then，the pipe needle is used for painless needle inserting （Fig. 3-9）. Taking the umbilicus as the center，the doctor performs radially horizontal needling at an angle of 10° outwardly. The depth of needle inserting is about 0.8 cun（Fig. 3-10）.

调气（图 3-11、图 3-12）。进针后嘱患者继续做腹式吐纳运动 3～5 分钟，直至感觉脐部出现温暖感。其间，如果患者身体的某个部位出现疼痛或其他不适，则提示该处三道两路受阻，需在痛点加刺 1 针。

Qi regulation（Fig. 3-11，Fig. 3-12）. The patient is instructed to continue the abdominal respiratory movement for 3 to 5 minutes after needle inserting until the patient feels the warmth of the umbilicus. If the patient feels pain or discomfort in some position，it means that three passages and two pathways are blocked，and one more needle inserting is required for this position.

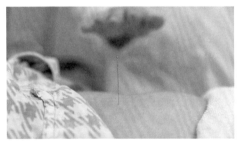 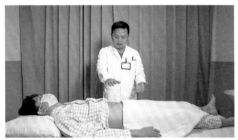

图 3-11　调气——近　　　　　　　　图 3-12　调气——远
Fig. 3-11　Qi regulation—short distance　　Fig. 3-12　Qi regulation—long distance

出针。嘱患者做腹式吐纳运动，趁患者吐气时，将针缓慢拔出。出针后立即用消毒棉签按压针孔，并轻轻揉压几次，防止气血外泄及出血。

Withdrawing the needle. The patient is instructed to perform abdominal respiratory movement，and then the doctor withdraws needles. The pinhole should be pressed with a sterile cotton swab immediately after the needle is withdrawn. Then，press the pinhole gently several times to prevent bleeding and the leakage of qi.

（6）施术后处理。检查针数量以防遗漏，用过的针具置于利器盒中销毁处理。

（6）Postoperative treatment. The number of needles should be checked to avoid omission. Besides，the used needles should be put in a sharps box for disposal.

（7）整理患者衣物及操作物品。

（7）The doctor tidies up the patient's clothing and used materials.

（8）交代患者治疗后注意事项等。

（8）The doctor informs the patient of precautions after treatment.

（9）洗手并记录治疗情况。

（9）The doctor washes hands and makes a record about treatment.

六、疗程
Ⅵ　Course of treatment

一般情况下留针时间为 30 分钟，可以依据患者情况进行灵活调整，延长留针时间至 30～50 分钟。视各类疾病不同，壮医针刺治疗疗程不同，急性病一般疗程短，通常每天针刺治疗 1 次，5～7 天为 1 个疗程；慢性病则疗程较长，可每天针刺治疗 1 次或隔天治疗 1 次，15～20 天为 1 个疗程。

In general，the time of prolonged needling for acu-esthesia is 30 minutes. Besides，the time of prolonged needling for acu-esthesia can be extended to 30 to 50 minutes according to the patient's disease condition. Zhuang medical course of acupuncture treatment varies because of different diseases. For acute diseases，the course of treatment is short（once a day，5 to 7 days as a course of treatment）. For chronic diseases，the course of treatment is long（once a day or once every two days，15 to 20 days as a course of treatment）.

七、注意事项
Ⅶ　Notes

（1）向患者耐心解释，说明壮医针灸主张无痛及在享受中治疗，以消除患者的紧张心理，令其放松心情，配合治疗。

（1）The doctor should explain to the patient that Zhuang medicine acupuncture advocates painless and comfortable treatment to help the patient overcome his/her nervousness and make him/her cooperate with the doctor for a better treatment.

（2）严格执行无菌操作。

（2）Aseptic operation should be strictly implemented.

（3）不宜取站立位治疗，以防患者晕针。

（3）It is not advisable to treat in an erect position in case of fainting during acupuncture.

（4）准确取穴，正确运用进针方法，掌握好进针的角度和深度。

（4）Acupoints should be selected correctly and the needle inserting method should be used rightly. Besides，the doctor should control the angle and depth of the needle inserting.

（5）针刺中应观察患者面色、神情，询问其有无不适反应，了解患者心理、生理感受，如发现病情变化，应立即对症处理。

（5）The doctor should observe the patient's complexion and expression，inquiry his/her discomfort to understand his/her feeling. If there are some changes in the disease condition，the doctor should immediately implement symptomatic treatment.

（6）起针时要核对穴位和针数，以免毫针遗留在患者身上。

（6）The number of acupoints and needles should be checked after the needles are withdrawn in case the filiform needles are left on the patient.

八、意外情况及处理
Ⅷ　Accidents and handling methods

（1）晕针。

（1）Fainting.

①症状。轻度晕针，表现为精神疲倦、头晕目眩、恶心欲吐；重度晕针，表现为心慌气短、面色苍白、出冷汗、脉象细弱，甚则神志昏迷、唇甲青紫、血压下降、二便失禁、脉微欲绝。

① Symptoms. The main manifestations of mild fainting during acupuncture are tiredness，dizziness and nausea. The main manifestations of severe fainting during acupuncture are palpitation and shortness of breath，pale complexion，cold sweating，thready pulse，even unconsciousness，cyanotic lips and nails，decreased blood pressure，urinary and fecal incontinence as well as barely palpable pulse.

②处理。立即停止针刺，取出所有留置针，让患者头低位平卧，亦可加服少量糖水；若出现严重至昏迷不醒者，立即行急救处理。

② Handling methods. The acupuncture should be stopped and all needles should be withdrawn immediately. Help the patient lie flat with head-down tilt and drink a small amount of sugar water. If the patient is unconscious，an emergency treatment should be performed immediately.

（2）滞针。

（2）Stuck needle.

①症状。针刺入穴位内因局部肌肉强烈收缩，或因行针时捻转角度过大、过快或持续单向捻转等，而致肌纤维缠绕针，运针时捻转不动，提插、出针均感困难。若勉强捻转、提插，则患者感到疼痛。

① Symptoms. Because of the intense contraction of local muscles，the large angle and fast speed of twirling the needle，or twirling the needle in one direction，needle inserting leads to the fact that the muscular fibers wrap around the needle and the doctor feels it difficult to twirl，lift，thrust and withdraw the needle. If the doctor twirls，lifts，thrusts or withdraws the needle in this situation，the patient will feel pain.

②处理。嘱患者消除紧张情绪，使局部肌肉放松，延长留针时间，用循、捏、按、弹等手法，或在滞针附近加刺针，以缓解局部肌肉紧张。如为单向捻针而致滞针者，需反向将针捻回。

② Handling methods. The patient is instructed to relax. Then，the doctor extends the time of prolonged needling，uses massage along meridian，pinching，pressing，plucking manipulation or adds a needle near the stuck needle to relieve the nervousness of local muscles. If the needle is twirled in one direction，the needle must be twirled back in the opposite direction.

（3）弯针。

（3）Bent needle.

①症状。针柄改变了进针时刺入的方向和角度，使提插、捻转和出针均感困难，患者感到针处疼痛。

① Symptom. The needle handle changes the direction and the angle of the needle-inserting, which makes the doctor feel it difficult to twirl, lift, thrust or withdraw the needle and the patient feel pain.

②处理。不能再行手法，如针身轻度弯曲，可慢慢将针退出；若弯曲角度过大，应顺着弯曲方向将针退出。因患者体位改变致弯针者，应嘱患者慢慢恢复原来体位，使局部肌肉放松后再慢慢退针。遇弯针时，切忌强拔针、猛退针。

② Handling methods. Stop this therapy. If the needle is slightly bent, the needle can be slowly withdrawn. If the bending angle is too large, the needle should be withdrawn along the bending direction. If it is caused by the change of the patient's posture, the doctor should help the patient to slowly restore the original posture. Then, the doctor slowly withdraws the needle after the patient relaxes the local muscles. In this case, it is prohibited to withdraw the needle with force.

（4）断针。

（4）Needle breakage.

①症状。针身折断，残端留于患者体内。

① Symptom. The needle body is broken, and a part of the needle is left in the patient's body.

②处理。嘱患者不要紧张、乱动，以防断针陷入深层。如残端显露，可用手指或镊子取出。若断端与皮肤相平，可用手指挤压针孔两旁，使断针暴露出体外，用镊子取出。如断针完全没入皮内、肌肉内，应在X线下定位，通过手术取出。

② Handling methods. The patient is instructed not to feel nervous or move to prevent the broken needle from going deeper into the body. If the broken part is exposed, the doctor can take it out with fingers or forceps. If the broken part is parallel with the skin, the doctor can squeeze the two sides of the pinhole with fingers until the broken end is exposed, then take it out with forceps. If the broken part completely enters the skin and muscle, X-ray positioning should be used to find out the exact location of the broken part. Then, the doctor takes it out through surgery.

（5）创伤性气胸。

（5）Traumatic pneumothorax.

①症状。患者突感胸闷、胸痛、气短、心悸，严重者呼吸困难、紫绀、出冷汗、烦躁、恐惧，甚则血压下降，出现休克等危急现象。检查时，患者肋间隙变宽、外胀，叩诊呈鼓声，听诊肺呼吸音减弱或消失。X线胸透可见肺组织被压缩现象，气管可向健侧移位。有的针刺创伤性轻度气胸者，起针后并不出现症状，而是过了一定时间才慢慢感到胸闷、胸痛、呼吸困难等。

① Symptoms. The patient suddenly develops signs of chest distress, chest pain, shortness of breath, palpitations, dyspnea, cyanosis, cold sweating, irritability, fear, even decreased blood pressure, shock, etc. During the examination, the intercostal space is widened and expanded and hyperresonant can be heard by percussion. Besides, the doctor can hear the lung breath sound is diminishing or disappearing by auscultation. X-ray shows that the lung tissue is compressed, and the trachea can be pulled towards the contralateral side. Some patients with mild traumatic pneumothorax have no symptoms after the needle is withdrawn but suffer from chest distress, chest pain, dyspnea and have other symptoms after a certain period.

②处理。一旦发生气胸，应立即起针，并让患者采取半卧位休息，嘱患者不要紧张，切勿因恐惧而翻转体位。一般漏气量少者，可自然吸收。医者要密切观察，随时对症处理，对症状严重患者须及时组织抢救。

② Handling methods. Once pneumothorax happens, the needle should be withdrawn immediately, and help the patient rest in semireclining position. The doctor should tell the patient not to be nervous or change posture in fear. In general, patients with mild pneumothorax will get spontaneous cure. The doctor should pay attention to the patient and take symptomatic treatment at any time. Besides, patients who have severe symptons must be rescued timely.

【附注】
【Notes】

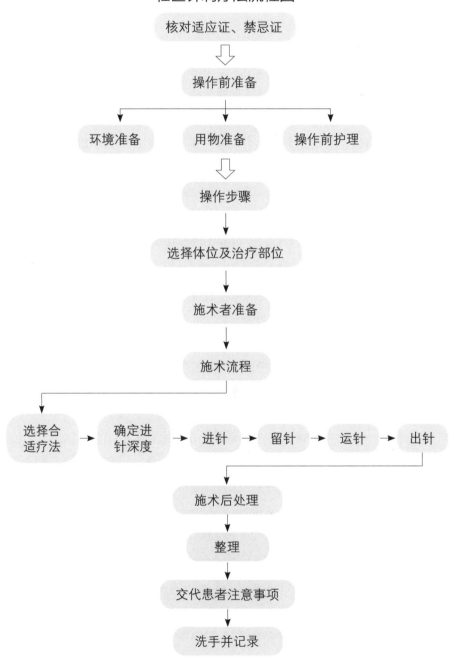

壮医针刺疗法流程图

The Flow Chart about Zhuang Medicine Acupuncture Therapy

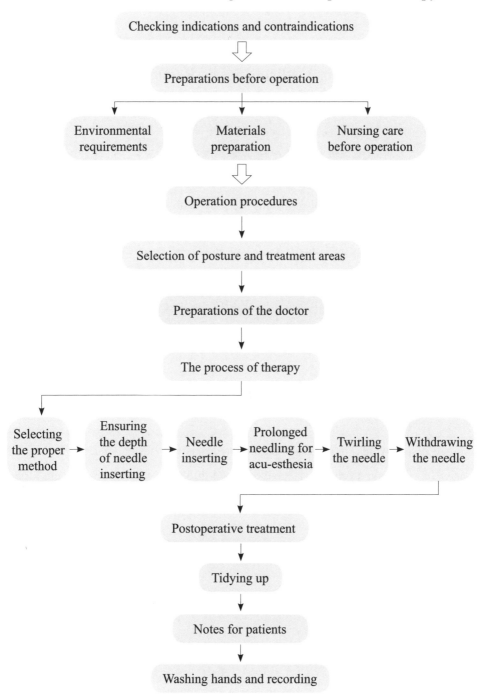

第四章　壮医莲花针拔罐逐瘀疗法
Chapter 4　Zhuang Medicine Stasis-Removing Therapy with Lotus-Needling and Cupping

　　壮医莲花针拔罐逐瘀疗法是在壮医独特理论的指导下，将莲花针叩刺与拔罐结合使用，以治疗疾病的一种方法，属于壮医针刺法的一种。

　　Zhuang medicine stasis-removing therapy with lotus-needling and cupping refers to a therapeutic method that combines the lotus-needling with cupping under the guidance of the unique theory of Zhuang medicine to remove stasis and subordinates to Zhuang medicine acupuncture methods.

一、主要功效
Ⅰ　Main effects

　　祛风、湿、痧、瘴、热、痰、瘀等毒，活血，消肿，散结，通痹，止痛，通调三道两路，调节气血平衡。

　　To dispel wind, dampness, pathogen, miasma, fever, phlegm and blood stasis. To eliminate swelling, stagnation, and arthralgia spasm. To promote blood circulation and relieve pain. To regulate three passages and two pathways and the balance between qi and blood.

二、适应证
Ⅱ　Indications

　　内科、外科、妇科、儿科、五官科、皮肤科等常见病、多发病、疑难病均可使用本疗法治疗，常见适应证有贫痧（痧症）、发旺（痹病）、核嘎尹（腰腿痛）、活邀尹（颈椎病）、旁巴尹（肩周炎）、骆芡（骨性关节炎）、隆芡（痛风）、麻抹（麻木）、甭裆呷（半身不遂）、林得叮相（跌打损伤）、年闹诺（失眠）、巧尹（头痛）、唪呗啷（带状疱疹、带状疱疹后遗神经痛）、能啥累（瘙痒、湿疹）、叻仇（痤疮）、泵栾（脱发）等。

This therapy can be used to treat the common diseases, frequently-occurring diseases and difficult miscellaneous diseases of internal medicine, surgery, gynecology, pediatrics, ENT, dermatology, etc. Its common indications are Pinsha（acute filthy disease）, Fawang（arthralgia disease）, Hegayin（lumbocrural pain）, Huoyaoyin（cervical spondylosis）, Pangbayin（scapulohumeral periarthritis）, Luoqian（osteoarthritis）, Longqian（gout）, Mamo（numbness）, Bengdangxia（hemiplegia）, Lindedingxiang（traumatic injury）, Niannaonuo（insomnia）, Qiaoyin（headache）, Benbeilang（shingles, postherpetic neuralgia）, Nenghanlei（pruritus, eczema）, Lechou（acne）, Bengluan（alopecia）, etc.

三、禁忌证
Ⅲ　Contraindications

（1）患自发出血性疾病、凝血功能障碍者禁用。

（1）It is prohibited for patients who have spontaneous hemorrhagic diseases and coagulation disorders.

（2）严重心脑血管疾病患者、血糖控制不佳者、精神病患者、身体极度消瘦虚弱者等禁用。

（2）It is prohibited for patients who have severe cardiovascular and cerebrovascular diseases, poor glycemic control, psychosis, or an extremely weak constitution.

（3）局部皮肤有破溃、疤痕、高度水肿处及浅表大血管处禁用。

（3）It is prohibited for patients who suffer from skin ulcers, scars and severe edema as well as superficial large vessels.

（4）过度疲劳、过度饥饿、过度饱或精神高度紧张的患者禁用。

（4）It is prohibited for patients who suffer from excessive fatigue, excessive hunger, overeating or high mental stress.

（5）孕妇禁用。

（5）It is prohibited for pregnant women.

四、操作前准备
Ⅳ　Preparations before operation

（1）环境要求。治疗室内清洁，安静，光线明亮，温度适宜，避免患者吹风受凉。

（1）Environmental requirements. The treatment room should be clean, quiet, well-lit. Besides, keep the treatment room at an ideal temperature to prevent the patient from catching a cold.

（2）用物准备。一次性莲花针（单头或双头皮肤针）（图4-1）、消毒真空抽气罐及真空抽气枪（图4-2）、复合碘皮肤消毒液、医用棉签、无菌纱布、镊子、一次性无菌手套、大毛巾、治疗车等。

（2）Materials preparation. A disposable lotus needle（single- or double-ended skin needle）（Fig. 4-1）, disinfected vacuum air suction cups and a vacuum air suction gun（Fig. 4-2）, compound iodine skin disinfectant, medical cotton swabs, sterile gauzes, forceps, disposable sterile gloves, large towels, a treatment cart, etc.

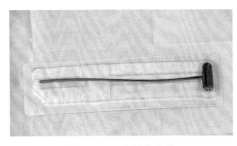

图 4-1　一次性莲花针
Fig. 4-1　A disposable lotus needle

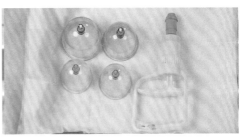

图 4-2　消毒真空抽气罐及真空抽气枪
Fig. 4-2　Disinfected vacuum air suction cups and a vacuum air suction gun

（3）操作前护理。核对患者信息及治疗方案等，说明治疗的意义和注意事项，取得患者同意；对患者进行精神安慰与鼓励，消除患者的紧张、恐惧情绪，使患者能积极主动配合操作。

（3）Nursing care before operation. The nurse should check the patient's information and treatment plan, explain the significance and notices of the treatment to obtain the patient's consent. Besides, the nurse should encourage the patient to overcome his/her nervousness and fear and enable the patient to cooperate with the doctor for a better operation.

五、操作步骤
V　Operation procedures

（1）体位选择。根据患者病情确定体位，常取坐位、俯卧位、仰卧位、侧卧位等，以患者舒适及便于施术者操作为宜，避免用强迫体位。

（1）Posture selection. Based on the state of the illness, the posture is selected. Sitting position, prone position, dorsal position or lateral recumbent position is often selected to provide convenience for the patient and the doctor. The compulsive position should be avoided.

（2）部位选择。常分为3类：循路，即依龙路、火路循行路线叩打（图4-3）；循点，即根据龙路、火路网结穴位的主治病症进行叩刺，常用于各种特定穴、反应点等（图4-4）；局部，即取局部病变部位进行围刺、散刺，常用于局部瘀肿疼痛、瘙痒、顽癣等（图4-5）。注意避开浅表大血管。

（2）Position selection. It is divided into three types：Tapping along the routes such as the dragon route（qi and blood route）and the fire route（sense route）（Fig. 4-3）；Tapping along the acupoints on the routes such as the dragon route and the fire route, which are commonly used in various specific acupoints, reaction points, etc.（Fig. 4-4）；Tapping along the local lesion sites, which is commonly used for local bruising, pain, itching, and psoriasis（Fig. 4-5）. Superficial large vessels should be avoided.

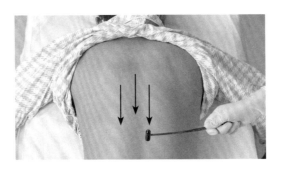

图 4-3 循路

Fig. 4-3 Tapping along the dragon route and the fire route

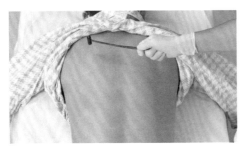

图 4-4 循点

Fig. 4-4 Tapping along the acupoints on the dragon route and the fire route

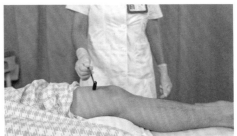

图 4-5 局部

Fig. 4-5 Tapping along the local lesion sites

（3）洗手，戴医用外科口罩、医用帽子和一次性无菌手套。

（3）The doctor should wash hands，wear a surgical mask，a medical cap and disposable sterile gloves.

（4）消毒。

（4）Disinfection.

①针具消毒。选择一次性莲花针。

① Needle disinfection. A disposable lotus needle is selected.

②部位消毒。常规消毒施术部位皮肤，消毒范围直径大于施术部位 5 cm（图 4-6）。

② Skin disinfection. The related skin is disinfected，and the diameter of the disinfection area is larger than that of treatment areas（exceeding 5 cm）（Fig. 4-6）.

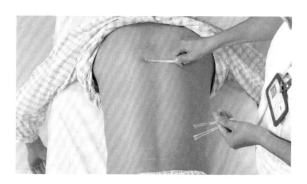

图 4-6　部位消毒

Fig. 4-6　Skin disinfection

（5）施术流程。

（5）Operation procedures.

①叩刺。右手握莲花针针柄尾部，食指在下，拇指在上（图 4-7），针尖对准叩刺部位，用腕力借助针柄弹性将针尖垂直叩打在皮肤上（图 4-8、图 4-9），反复进行，叩刺至皮肤微微渗血（图 4-10）。

① Needle tapping. The right hand holds the tail of the lotus needle handle with index finger and thumb，index finger above and thumb below the handle（Fig. 4-7）. Then，the doctor vertically taps related treatment area by the flexion movement of wrist and the elasticity of needle handle（Fig. 4-8，Fig. 4-9）and repeats it until the skin slightly oozes blood（Fig. 4-10）.

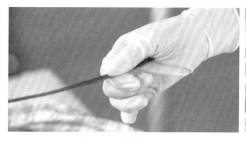

图 4-7　持针手法

Fig. 4-7　Needle holding manipulation

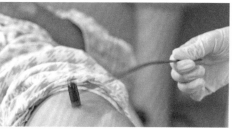

图 4-8　叩刺

Fig. 4-8　Needle tapping

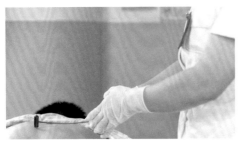 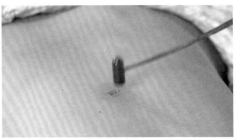

图 4-9　叩刺

Fig. 4-9　Needle tapping

图 4-10　皮肤微微渗血

Fig. 4-10　Slightly oozing blood from skin

②施罐。

② Cupping operation.

拔罐。叩刺完毕，左手将真空抽气罐扣压在叩刺部位，右手持真空抽气枪连接真空抽气罐气嘴进行抽气（图 4-11），使罐内形成负压。抽气次数以患者耐受为度。然后撤枪，给患者盖上大毛巾，留罐 10 ～ 15 分钟。

Cupping. The vacuum air suction cup held in the left hand is put on the treatment area after needle tapping, and the vacuum air suction gun held in the right hand is connected to the nozzle of the vacuum air suction cup to extract the air from the cup（Fig. 4-11）. Thus, negative pressure is formed in the cup. The number of air extraction is determined by the patient's feeling. Then the vacuum air suction gun is removed, and the patient is covered with a large towel. The cup needs to be kept for 10 to 15 minutes.

起罐。将真空抽气罐活塞拔起，然后把罐向一侧倾斜，让空气进入罐内，同时让瘀血流入罐内，慢慢将罐提起，用无菌纱布擦拭所拔部位流出的瘀血（图 4-12），常规消毒治疗部位的皮肤。

Removal of the cup. The doctor pulls up the piston of the vacuum air suction cup, tilts the cup to one side, lets the air and the blood stasis flow into the cup, then slowly lifts the cup and cleans the blood at treatment areas with sterile gauzes （Fig. 4-12）and the skin at this area is routinely disinfected.

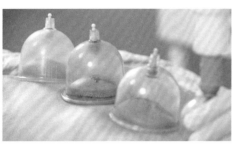
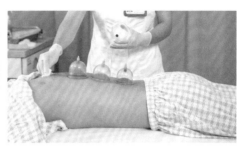

图 4-11　抽气

Fig. 4-11　Air extraction

图 4-12　擦拭

Fig. 4-12　Cleaning

（6）施术后处理。莲花针一人一针，用后丢入利器盒（图4-13）。冲洗真空抽气罐内瘀血并放入含氯消毒液中浸泡后送消毒供应中心统一消毒，防止交叉感染。

（6）Postoperative treatment. The lotus needle is disposable and should be thrown into the sharps box（Fig. 4-13）. The blood stasis in the vacuum air suction cup is cleaned and put in chlorine-containing disinfectant，and then sent to central sterile supply department to prevent cross infection.

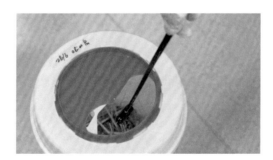

图 4-13　把莲花针丢入利器盒

Fig. 4-13　Throwing the lotus needle into the sharps box

（7）整理患者衣物及操作物品。

（7）The doctor tidies up the patient's clothing and used materials.

（8）交代患者治疗后注意事项等。

（8）The doctor informs the patient of precautions after treatment.

（9）洗手并记录治疗情况。

（9）The doctor washes hands and makes a record about treatment.

六、疗程

Ⅵ Course of treatment

隔天 1 次，10 次为 1 个疗程。

Once every other day，10 times as a course of treatment.

七、注意事项

Ⅶ Notes

（1）患者过度疲劳、过度饥饿、过度饱或精神高度紧张时不能操作。暴露治疗部位时，应注意保护患者隐私及保暖。

（1）It is prohibited for patients who suffer from excessive fatigue，excessive hunger，overeating or high mental stress. When treatment areas are exposed，the doctor should protect the patient's privacy and keep the patient warm.

（2）注意检查莲花针针尖，应平齐、无钩、无锈蚀和无缺损。

（2）Pay attention to checking the tip of lotus needle which should be straight and have no hook，rust or defect.

（3）叩打时，针尖应垂直，避免勾挑，叩刺范围应小于所选的罐号罐口。

（3）The tip of lotus needle should be perpendicular to treatment areas to avoid prick and the diameter of tapping area should be smaller than that of rim of selected cup.

（4）根据患者的病情及施术部位选择相应规格的皮肤针。叩刺手法分为轻手法、重手法和中手法 3 种。轻手法为轻腕力叩刺，以局部皮肤潮红为宜，适用于老弱者、头面部等肌肉浅薄处；重手法以较重腕力敲打叩刺，至局部皮肤隐隐出血为宜，用于壮者、实证及肌肉丰厚处；中手法介于轻手法与重手法之间，以局部皮肤潮红、局部无渗血为宜，适用于一般疾病及多数患者。

（4）According to the patient's disease condition and treatment area，the corresponding skin needles are selected. Needle tapping manipulations are divided into mild，moderate and intense manipulation. The mild manipulation refers to needle tapping with mild wrist force. It is featured by local skin flushing and is suitable for the elderly and the patients with weak constitution, and the treatment areas with thin muscles such as head, face, etc. The intense manipulation refers to needle tapping with intense wrist force. It is featured by local oozing of blood, and is suitable for the patients with strong constitution, excess syndrome and the treatment areas with thick muscles. The moderate manipulation is between mild and intense manipulations. It is featured by local skin flushing and no oozing of blood and is suitable for common diseases and most patients.

（5）治疗过程中随时观察患者局部皮肤及病情，随时询问患者对叩刺及施罐的耐受程度，防止患者晕针、晕罐。

（5）During this process, the doctor should observe the patient's skin and condition as well as ask the patient's tolerance to this therapy at any time in case of fainting during acupuncture and cupping.

（6）治疗过程中应遵守无菌操作规则，防止感染。

（6）Aseptic operation should be obeyed during the treatment to prevent infection.

（7）治疗后避免患者立即起身离开，为其安排舒适的体位，并嘱其休息5～10分钟后方可活动。

（7）Prevent the patient from getting up and leaving immediately after treatment. Let the patient take a comfortable posture and rest for 5 to 10 minutes.

（8）施术后交代患者，若施术部位有瘙痒，属正常的治疗反应，避免用手抓破，以免引起感染；保持施术部位皮肤清洁干燥，6小时内不宜淋浴。

（8）The patient should be instructed that itching on the treatment areas is a normal treatment reaction, do not scratch it in case of infection, keep the skin of treatment areas clean and dry. Besides, it is not suitable to take a shower within 6 hours after treatment.

（9）治疗后在饮食上应注意忌口，以清淡饮食为主。

（9）Diet should be paid attention to after the treatment. The patient should eat on a bland diet during treatment.

八、意外情况及处理
VIII　Accidents and handling methods

（1）晕针、晕罐。如患者治疗过程中出现气短、面色苍白、出冷汗等晕针现象，立即让患者头低位平卧，亦可加服少量糖水；若出现严重至昏迷不醒者，立即行急救处理。

（1）Fainting. If the patient develops shortness of breath，pale complexion and cold sweat during treatment，this operation should be stopped immediately，and help the patient lie flat with head-down tilt and drink a small amount of sugar water. If the patient is unconscious，an emergency treatment should be performed immediately.

（2）烫伤、起水疱。如有烫伤，用生理盐水清洁创面并浸润无菌纱布湿敷创面直至疼痛明显减轻或消失后，外涂烧伤膏。如起小水疱，皮肤可自行吸收，保持局部干燥及水疱皮肤的完整性即可；如水疱较大，可用无菌针头将水疱戳破，放出疱内渗液，每日用碘伏消毒，外涂烧伤膏，保持局部干燥及清洁，预防感染。

（2）Scalds and blisters. For scalds，the surface of the wound should be cleaned with physiological saline and compressed by wet sterile gauzes until the pain is greatly relieved or disappears，and then applied burn ointment. For small blisters，the skin will absorb the blisters fluid if the skin over the blisters is not open and kept dry. For large blisters，a sterile needle can be used to puncture them to release the fluid. Then disinfect it with iodophor，apply burn ointment to it，and keep the skin dry and clean every day to prevent infection.

【附注】
【Notes】

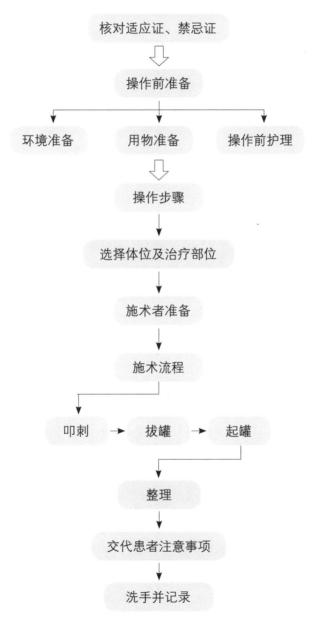

壮医莲花针拔罐逐瘀疗法流程图

核对适应证、禁忌证

操作前准备

环境准备　　　用物准备　　　操作前护理

操作步骤

选择体位及治疗部位

施术者准备

施术流程

叩刺　→　拔罐　→　起罐

整理

交代患者注意事项

洗手并记录

The Flow Chart about Zhuang Medicine Stasis-Removing Therapy with Lotus-Needling and Cupping

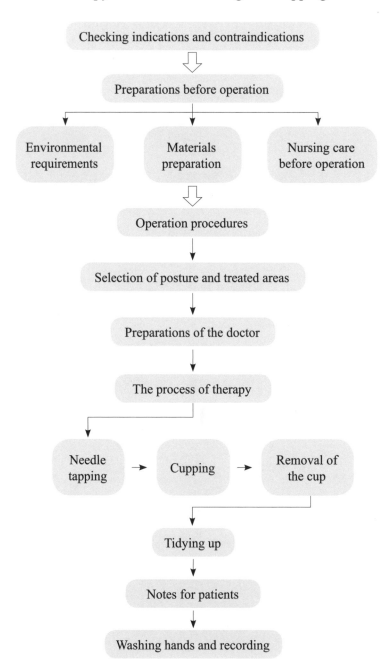

第五章　壮医刮痧疗法
Chapter 5　Zhuang Medicine Skin Scraping Therapy

壮医刮痧疗法是采用边缘光滑的牛角片、羊角片、嫩竹板、瓷片、动物骨、药材等工具，以刮痧油、药酒或凡士林等为介质，在体表部位进行反复刮拭，从而对机体产生良性刺激，以治疗和预防疾病的一种方法。

Zhuang medicine skin scraping therapy refers to a therapeutic method of taking horns，bamboo clappers，porcelain slices，animal bones and herbs which have smooth edge as tools and scraping oil，medicinal liquor and Vaseline as the medium to scrape the skin，which can produce a positive stimulus to the body.

一、主要功效
Ⅰ　Main effects

祛风、湿、痧、瘴、热、痰、瘀等毒，消肿，散结，通痹，通调三道两路，调节气血平衡。

To dispel wind，dampness，pathogen，miasma，fever，phlegm and blood stasis. To eliminate swelling，stagnation，and arthralgia spasm. To regulate three passages and two pathways and the balance between qi and blood.

二、适应证
Ⅱ　Indications

内科、外科、儿科、皮肤科、五官科等常见病、多发病均可使用本疗法治疗，常见适应证有贫痧（痧症）、发得（发热）、奔唉（咳嗽）、发旺（痹病）、甬巧尹（偏头痛）、巧尹（头痛）、活邀尹（颈椎病）、旁巴尹（肩周炎）、核嘎尹（腰腿痛）、麻抹（麻木）、甬裆呷（半身不遂）、年闹诺（失眠）、林得叮相（跌打损伤）、嚎尹（牙痛）、肥胖症等。

This therapy can be used to treat the common diseases and frequently-occurring diseases of internal medicine, surgery, pediatrics, dermatology, ENT, etc. Its common indications include Pinsha（acute filthy disease）, Fade（fever）, Ben'ai（cough）, Fawang（arthralgia disease）, Bengqiaoyin（migraine）, Qiaoyin（headache）, Huoyaoyin（cervical spondylosis）, Pangbayin（scapulohumeral periarthritis）, Hegayin（lumbocrural pain）, Mamo（numbness）, Bengdangxia（hemiplegia）, Niannaonuo（insomnia）, Lindedingxiang（traumatic injury）, Haoyin（toothache）, obesity, etc.

三、禁忌证
Ⅲ Contraindications

（1）自发出血性疾病患者、凝血功能障碍者禁用。

（1）It is prohibited for patients who have spontaneous hemorrhagic disease and coagulation disorders.

（2）严重心脑血管疾病患者、血糖控制不佳者、精神病患者、身体极度消瘦虚弱者等禁用。

（2）It is prohibited for patients who have severe cardiovascular and cerebrovascular diseases, poor glycemic control, psychosis, or an extremely weak constitution.

（3）刮治部位的皮肤有损伤及病变处禁用。

（3）It is prohibited for damaged skin and skin lesions.

（4）急性扭伤、创伤的疼痛部位或骨折部位禁用。

（4）It is prohibited for pain site or fracture site caused by acute sprain and trauma.

（5）孕妇的腹部、腰骶部，妇女的乳头禁用。

（5）It is prohibited for pregnant women's abdomen, lumbosacral portion and nipples.

（6）大病初愈、重病、气血亏虚者禁用。

（6）It is prohibited for patients recovering from serious illness，patients with severe illness，qi and blood deficiency.

（7）过度疲劳、过度饥饿、过度饱、精神高度紧张、饮酒后及对刮痧有恐惧者禁用。

（7）It is prohibited for patients who suffer from excessive fatigue，excessive hunger，overeating or high mental stress. Besides，it is also prohibited for patients drinking liquor or feeling fear to this therapy.

四、操作前准备
Ⅳ　Preparations before operation

（1）环境要求。治疗室内清洁，安静，光线明亮，温度适宜，避免患者吹风受凉。

（1）Environmental requirements. The treatment room should be clean，quiet，well-lit. Besides，keep the treatment room at an ideal temperature to prevent the patient from catching a cold.

（2）用物准备。刮痧板（图 5-1）、刮痧油（或药酒、凡士林等）（图 5-2）、治疗盘、治疗碗、75% 酒精、生理盐水、棉球、无菌纱布、治疗巾、一次性无菌手套。

（2）Materials preparation. Scraping plates（Fig. 5-1），scraping oil（or medicinal liquor，Vaseline，etc.）（Fig. 5-2），a medical tray，a treatment bowl，75% alcohol，physiological saline，cotton balls，sterile gauzes，treatment towels，disposable sterile gloves.

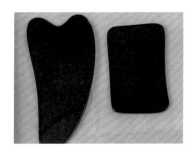

图 5-1　刮痧板
Fig. 5-1　Scraping plates

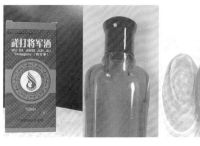

图 5-2　药酒、刮痧油、凡士林
Fig. 5-2　Medicinal liquor，scraping oil and Vaseline

（3）操作前护理。 核对患者信息及治疗方案等，说明治疗的意义和注意事项，取得患者同意；对患者进行精神安慰与鼓励，消除患者的紧张、恐惧情绪，使患者能积极主动配合操作。

（3）Nursing care before operation. The nurse should check the patient's information and treatment plan and explain the significance and notices of the treatment to obtain the patient's consent. Besides, the nurse should encourage the patient to overcome his/her nervousness and fear and enable the patient to cooperate with the doctor for a better operation.

五、操作步骤
V　Operation procedures

（1）体位选择。常取坐位、俯卧位、仰卧位、侧卧位等，根据患者病情确定体位，以患者舒适及便于施术者操作为宜，避免用强迫体位。

（1）Posture selection. Based on the state of the illness, the posture is selected. Sitting position, prone position, dorsal position or lateral recumbent position is often selected to provide convenience for the patient and the doctor. The compulsive position should be avoided.

（2）部位选择。根据病证选取适当的治疗部位。

（2）Position selection. According to the disease patterns, the corresponding treatment area is selected.

（3）洗手，戴医用外科口罩、医用帽子和一次性无菌手套。

（3）The doctor should wash hands, wear a surgical mask, a medical cap, and disposable sterile gloves.

（4）消毒。

（4）Disinfection.

①刮具消毒。用 75% 酒精消毒刮痧板（图 5-3）。

① Disinfection of scraping tools. Disinfect the scraping plate with 75% alcohol （Fig. 5-3）.

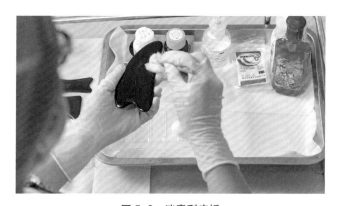

图 5-3　消毒刮痧板

Fig. 5-3　Disinfection of the scraping plate

②部位消毒。用生理盐水蘸棉球或无菌纱布清洁将要刮治部位的皮肤。

② Skin disinfection. Disinfect the skin of treatment area with the cotton balls or sterile gauzes with physiological saline.

（5）施术流程。

（5）Operation procedures.

①涂擦。将刮痧油（或药酒、凡士林等）倒入治疗碗内（图 5-4），用棉球或无菌纱布蘸刮痧油（或药酒、凡士林等）涂擦刮痧部位。

① Inunction. Poured scraping oil（or medicinal liquor，Vaseline，etc.）into the treatment bowl（Fig. 5-4）and inunct the scraping site with cotton balls or sterile gauzes dipping in scraping oil（or medicinal liquor，Vaseline，etc.）.

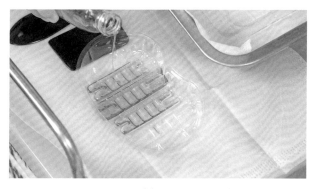

图 5-4　将刮痧油倒入治疗碗内

Fig. 5-4　Pouring scraping oil into the treatment bowl

②刮痧。施术者手拿刮痧板，刮痧板厚的一侧对着手掌（图5-5），用另一侧在患者体表治疗部位反复刮拭。整个身躯刮拭原则：从上到下（图5-6），从前到后，先中间后两边（图5-7）。刮拭要领：急者先喉，缓者顺受，肌肉骨节，近自远收。刮拭顺序为颈→背→腰→腹→上肢→下肢，从上向下刮拭，胸背部从内向外刮拭。刮痧板与刮拭方向一般保持45°～90°（图5-8），刮时要沿同一个方向刮，采用腕力，力量均匀。一般每个部位刮10～20次，时间3～5分钟，最长不超过20分钟，以皮肤出现紫色痧点为宜（图5-9）。

② Scraping. The doctor holds a scraping plate with the thick part facing the palm（Fig. 5-5）, and repeatedly scrapes treatment areas with the other part of the scraping plate. The scraping principle for the whole body: from top to bottom（Fig. 5-6）, from front to back, from middle to both sides（Fig. 5-7）. Key points of scraping: it should begin from top to bottom and from the near to the distant. The order of scraping is neck → back → waist → abdomen → upper limbs → lower limbs, from top to bottom, from inside to outside of chest and back. The angle between scraping plate and the scraping direction maintains at 45° to 90°（Fig. 5-8）. When scraping, the doctor should scrape in the same direction with steady wrist force. In general, scrape each treatment area 10 to 20 times which lasts 3 to 5 minutes. It should not last for more than 20 minutes. It is the best that the skin appears purple spots（Fig. 5-9）.

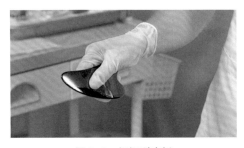

图 5-5　抓握刮痧板
Fig. 5-5　Holding the scraping plate

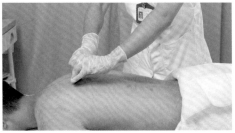

图 5-6　从上到下刮拭
Fig. 5-6　Scraping from top to bottom

（6）施术后处理。用无菌纱布清洁刮治部位皮肤（图5-10）（根据患者病情需要可在刮治部位涂擦药酒），洗净刮痧板，用75%酒精消毒刮痧板。

（6）Postoperative treatment. The skin of treatment area is cleaned with sterile gauzes（Fig. 5-10）（inunction of medicinal liquor to the scraping site according to the patient's disease condition）and the scraping plate is cleaned and disinfected with 75% alcohol.

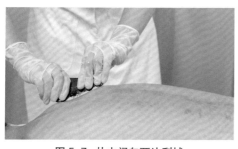

图 5-7　从中间向两边刮拭
Fig. 5-7　Scraping from middle to both sides

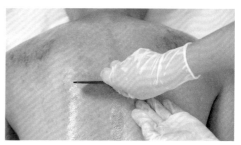

图 5-8　刮板与刮拭方向保持 45°～ 90°
Fig. 5-8　The angle between scraping plate and the scraping direction maintains at 45° to 90°

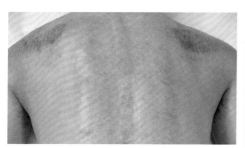

图 5-9　紫色痧点
Fig. 5-9　Purple spots

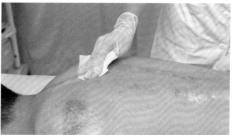

图 5-10　清洁皮肤
Fig. 5-10　Cleaning the skin

（7）整理患者衣物及操作物品。

（7）The doctor tidies up the patient's clothing and used materials.

（8）交代患者治疗后注意事项等。

（8）The doctor informs the patient of precautions after treatment.

（9）洗手并记录治疗情况。

（9）The doctor washes hands and makes a record about treatment.

六、疗程
Ⅵ　Course of treatment

根据患者病情而定。急性病证 1 ～ 2 天 1 次，慢性病证 3 ～ 5 天 1 次，5

次为1个疗程。

According to the patient's disease condition，this therapy can be performed once every 1 to 2 days for acute diseases，once every 3 to 5 days for chronic diseases and a course of treatment is 5 times.

七、注意事项
Ⅶ Notes

（1）患者过度疲劳、过度饥饿、过度饱、精神高度紧张、饮酒后及对刮痧有恐惧时不能操作。暴露治疗部位时，应注意保护患者隐私及保暖。

（1）It is prohibited for patients who suffer from excessive fatigue，excessive hunger，overeating or high mental stress. Besides，it is also prohibited for patients drinking liquor or feeling fear to this therapy. When treatment areas are exposed，the doctor should protect the patient's privacy and keep the patient warm.

（2）不能干刮，刮痧板必须边缘光滑、没有破损，以免刮伤患者皮肤。

（2）Scraping needs medium and the scraping plate should have smooth edges and no damage so as not to scratch the patient's skin.

（3）对于部分不出痧或痧点的患者，不可强求出痧或痧点，以患者感到舒适为宜。

（3）For some patients who have no purple or red spots，the doctor cannot continue the operation until purple or red spots occur on the skin. It is the most important that patients feel comfortable.

（4）年轻、体壮、新病、急病的实证患者用重刮，即刮拭按压力大、速度快。正常人保健或虚实兼见证患者用平补平泻法，即刮拭按压力中等、速度适中。正确选取刮拭部位，只有根据不同的病证选取相应的穴位刮痧，效果才会显著。

（4）Intense scraping is suitable for young patients，strong patients and patients with acute diseases，that is，scraping needs enough strength and fast speed. Neutral supplementation and draining method are suitable for normal people for health care or patients with excess and deficiency syndrome，that is，scraping needs appropriate strength and speed. Select the right scraping sites. Only in this way that the doctor selects the corresponding acupoints to scrape according to different diseases will the effect be significant.

（5）前一次刮痧部位的痧斑未退之前，不宜在原处再次进行刮痧。再次刮痧时间需间隔 3 ～ 6 天，以皮肤痧退为准。

（5）It is not advisable to perform scraping again on the original place before spots disappear. The time interval of scraping should be 3 to 6 days, which is based on spots' disappearance.

（6）治疗过程中随时观察患者局部皮肤及病情，随时询问患者的耐受程度，防止患者晕刮。

（6）During this process, the doctor should observe the patient's skin and condition as well as ask the patient's tolerance to this therapy at any time.

（7）治疗后避免患者立即起身离开，为其安排舒适的体位，给患者饮一杯温开水，并嘱其休息 15 ～ 20 分钟后方可活动。

（7）Prevent the patient from getting up and leaving immediately after treatment. Let the patient drink a cup of warm water, take a comfortable posture and rest for 15 to 20 minutes.

（8）告知患者，刮痧部位会有疼痛、灼热感，属于正常现象；刮痧部位出现红紫色痧点或瘀斑，数日后方可消失，不必害怕；刮痧后 4 小时内忌洗澡，刮痧部位注意保暖，避免吹风受寒。

（8）The patient is instructed that there is pain and burning sensation in the scraping areas, which is normal. Red and purple spots or ecchymosis may appear in the scraping areas, which can disappear in a few days. Do not take a bath with 4 hours after the scraping. The scraping areas should be kept warm to avoid catching a cold.

（9）治疗后在饮食上注意忌口，以清淡饮食为主。

（9）Diet should be paid attention to after the treatment. The patient should be on a bland diet during treatment.

八、意外情况及处理

VIII　Accidents and handling methods

（1）晕刮。如患者治疗过程中出现气短、面色苍白、出冷汗等现象，立即让患者头低位平卧，亦可加服少量糖水；若出现严重至昏迷不醒者，立即行急救处理。

（1）Fainting. If the patient develops shortness of breath, pale complexion and cold sweat during treatment, this operation should be stopped immediately, and help the patient lie flat with head-down tilt and drink a small amount of sugar water. If the patient is unconscious, an emergency treatment should be performed immediately.

（2）刮伤、起水疱。如有刮伤，用生理盐水清洁创面并浸润无菌纱布湿敷创面直至疼痛明显减轻或消失后，外涂烧伤膏。如局部皮肤起小水疱，皮肤可自行吸收，保持局部干燥及水疱皮肤的完整性即可，预防感染。

（2）Scratches and blisters. For scratches, the surface of the wound should be cleaned with physiological saline and compressed by wet sterile gauzes until the pain is greatly relieved or disappears, and then applied burn ointment. For small blisters, the skin will absorb the blisters fluid if the skin over the blisters is not open and kept dry to prevent infection.

【附注】
【Notes】

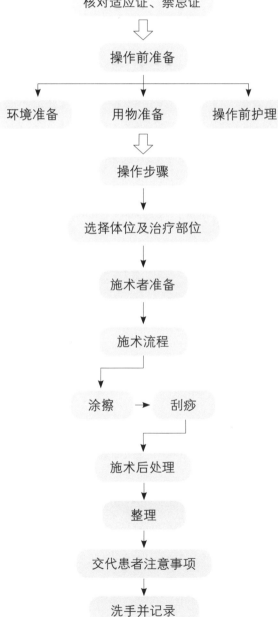

壮医刮痧疗法流程图

核对适应证、禁忌证

操作前准备

环境准备　　用物准备　　操作前护理

操作步骤

选择体位及治疗部位

施术者准备

施术流程

涂擦　→　刮痧

施术后处理

整理

交代患者注意事项

洗手并记录

The Flow Chart about Zhuang Medicine Skin Scraping Therapy

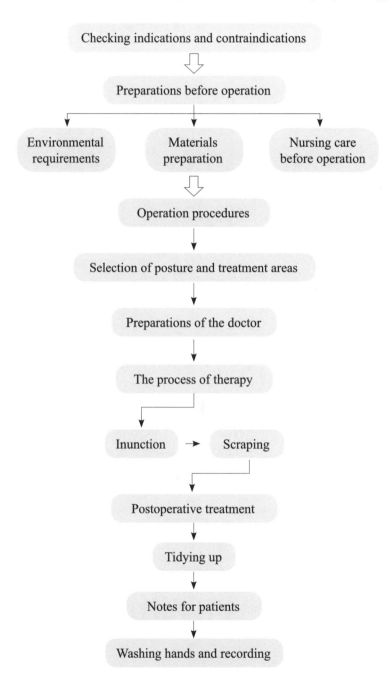

第六章　壮医烫熨疗法
Chapter 6　Zhuang Medicine Ironing Therapy

壮医烫熨疗法是将壮药装入纱布袋后放入煮沸的水中蒸热，趁热将药包直接熨于患处，加以手法反复烫熨，利用其药力、热力治疗疾病的一种方法。

Zhuang medicine ironing therapy refers to a therapeutic method of putting Zhuang medicinal materials into the gauze bag, steaming it with boiling water, and then repeatedly ironing treatment areas with the herbal medicinals and heat to treat diseases.

一、主要功效
Ⅰ　Main effects

祛风、湿、瘴、寒、痰、瘀等毒，消肿，散结，通痹，止痛，通调三道两路，调节气血平衡。

To dispel wind, dampness, miasma, cold, phlegm and blood stasis. To eliminate swelling, stagnation, arthralgia spasm and pain. To regulate three passages and two pathways and the balance between qi and blood.

二、适应证
Ⅱ　Indications

内科、外科、妇科、儿科、皮肤科等常见病、多发病均可使用本疗法治疗，常见适应证有核嘎尹（腰腿痛）、活邀尹（颈椎病）、旁巴尹（肩周炎）、麻抹（麻木）、林得叮相（跌打损伤）、发旺（痹病）、隆芡（痛风）、嗉佛（包块肿块）、嗉尹（疼痛）、嗉呗嘟（带状疱疹、带状疱疹后遗神经痛）、腊胴尹（腹痛）、京尹（痛经）、约京乱（月经不调）、卟很裆（不孕）、盆腔炎、屙细（泄泻）、北嘻（乳腺炎）等。

This therapy can be used to treat the common diseases and frequently-occurring diseases of internal medicine，surgery，gynecology，pediatrics，dermatology，etc. Its common indications include Hegayin（lumbocrural pain），Huoyaoyin（cervical spondylosis），Pangbayin（scapulohumeral periarthritis），Mamo（numbness），Lindedingxiang（traumatic injury），Fawang（arthralgia disease），Longqian（gout），Benfo（lump），Benyin（pain），Benbeilang（shingles，postherpetic neuralgia），Ladongyin（abdominal pain），Jingyin（dysmenorrhea），Yuejingluan（irregular menstruation），Buhendang（infertility），pelvic inflammatory disease，Exi（diarrhea），Beixi（mastitis），etc.

三、禁忌证
Ⅲ　Contraindications

（1）辨证为阳证患者禁用。

（1）It is prohibited for patients with Yang syndrome.

（2）发热（体温≥37.3 ℃）、脉搏≥90次/分患者禁用。

（2）It is prohibited for patients with fever（body temperature ≥ 37.3 ℃）or pulse rate ≥ 90 beats/min.

（3）有开放性创口或感染性病灶者禁用。

（3）It is prohibited for patients with open wounds or infectious lesions.

（4）过度疲劳、过度饥饿、过度饱或精神高度紧张的患者禁用。

（4）It is prohibited for patients who suffer from excessive fatigue，excessive hunger，overeating or high mental stress.

（5）严重心脑血管疾病患者、血糖控制不佳者、精神病患者、身体极度消瘦虚弱者等禁用。

（5）It is prohibited for patients who have severe cardiovascular and cerebrovascular diseases，poor glycemic control，psychosis，or an extremely weak constitution.

（6）孕妇禁用。

（6）It is prohibited for pregnant women.

四、操作前准备
Ⅳ　Preparations before operation

（1）环境要求。治疗室内清洁，安静，光线明亮，温度适宜，避免患者吹风受凉。

（1）Environmental requirements. The treatment room should be clean, quiet, well-lit. Besides, keep the treatment room at an ideal temperature to prevent the patient from catching a cold.

（2）用物准备。

（2）Materials preparation.

①一次性无菌手套、纱布袋（图6-1）、防烫厚胶手套（图6-2）、防水垫巾、消毒毛巾、一次性治疗巾。

① Disposable sterile gloves, a gauze bag（Fig. 6-1）, anti-scalding rubber gloves（Fig. 6-2）, a waterproof towel, disinfected towels, a disposable treatment towels.

②药物。根据患者病情选择相应已用特制药酒浸泡过的壮药，将其装入纱布袋（图6-3），放入煮沸的水中蒸热30分钟（图6-4）。

② Herbs. According to the patient's disease condition, Zhuang medicinal materials that have been soaked in the medicinal liquor is put into the gauze bag（Fig. 6-3）, and then steamed in the boiling water for 30 minutes（Fig. 6-4）.

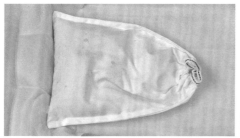

图6-1　纱布袋
Fig. 6-1　Gauze bag

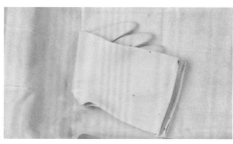

图6-2　防烫厚胶手套
Fig. 6-2　Anti-scalding rubber gloves

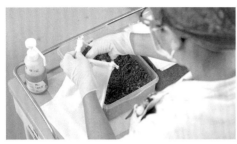

图 6-3　装药入袋

Fig. 6-3　Putting the herbs in the bag

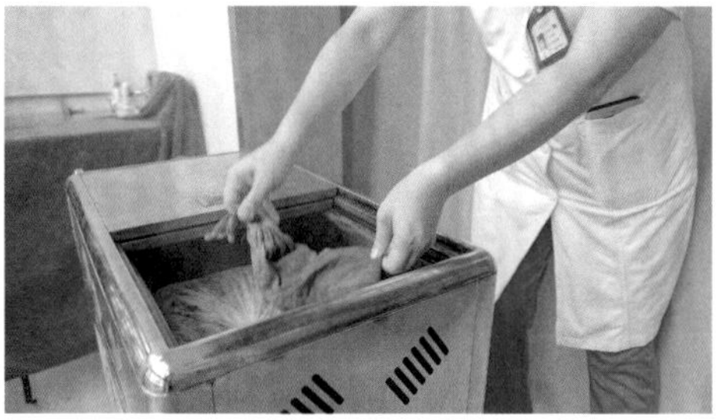

图 6-4　蒸煮药袋

Fig. 6-4　Steaming the bag filled with herbs

（3）操作前护理。核对患者信息及治疗方案等，说明治疗的意义和注意事项，并取得患者同意；对患者进行精神安慰与鼓励，消除患者的紧张、恐惧情绪，使患者能积极主动配合操作。

（3）Nursing care before operation. The nurse should check the patient's information and treatment plan and explain the significance and notices of the treatment to obtain the patient's consent. Besides, the nurse should encourage the patient to overcome his/her nervousness and fear and enable the patient to cooperate with the doctor for a better operation.

五、操作步骤
V　Operation procedures

（1）体位选择。根据患者病情确定体位，常取坐位、俯卧位、仰卧位、侧卧位等，以患者舒适及便于施术者操作为宜，避免用强迫体位。

（1）Posture selection. Based on the state of illness, the posture is selected. Sitting position, prone position, dorsal position or lateral recumbent position is often selected to provide convenience for the patient and the doctor. The compulsive position should be avoided.

（2）部位选择。根据病证选取适当的治疗部位。

（2）Position selection. According to the disease patterns, the corresponding treatment area is selected.

（3）洗手，戴医用外科口罩、医用帽子和一次性无菌手套，最外层戴防烫厚胶手套。

（3）The doctor should wash hands，wear a surgical mask，a medical cap，disposable sterile gloves and anti-scalding rubber gloves.

（4）施术流程。

（4）Operation procedures.

①悬熨。将药熨包悬在治疗部位上方作快速环形移动（图 6-5）。

① Ironing with the way of suspending. The bag filled with herbs is suspended and moved rapidly above treatment areas（Fig. 6-5）.

②点熨。将药熨包由内向外快速垂直点烫治疗部位（图 6-6）。

② Ironing with the way of stinging. Treatment areas are ironed vertically and rapidly from inside to outside with the bag filled with herbs（Fig. 6-6）.

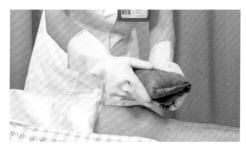 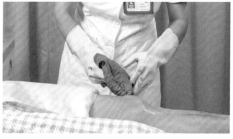

图 6-5　悬熨 　　　　　　　　　　　　图 6-6　点熨

Fig. 6-5　Ironing with the way of suspending　　　Fig. 6-6　Ironing with the way of stinging

③按熨。将药熨包按压于治疗部位，使之与皮肤接触面积增大（图 6-7）。

③ Ironing with the way of pressing. The bag filled with herbs is pressed on treatment areas to increase the skin contact area（Fig. 6-7）.

④揉熨。持药熨包用力揉按治疗部位，速度稍慢，力度加大（图 6-8）。

④ Ironing with the way of kneading. Treatment areas are kneaded vigorously and slowly with the bag filled with herbs（Fig. 6-8）.

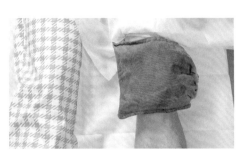

图 6-7 按熨

Fig. 6-7　Ironing with the way of pressing

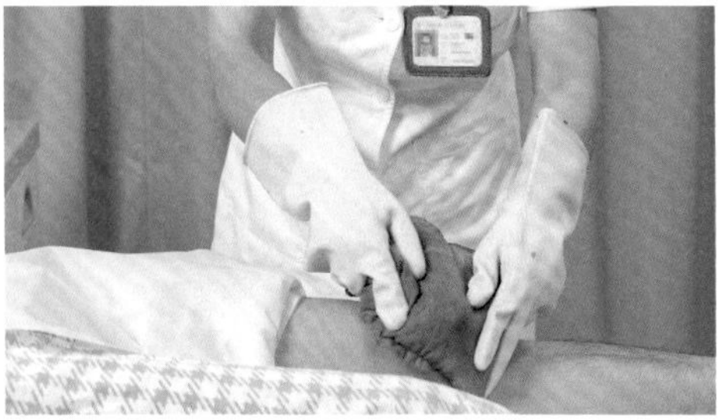

图 6-8 揉熨

Fig. 6-8　Ironing with the way of kneading

⑤敷熨。将还有余温的药熨包敷在治疗部位，盖上防水垫巾及一次性治疗巾，使药力进一步渗透，保持 10 ～ 15 分钟（图 6-9）。

⑤ Ironing with the way of compressing. The bag filled with herbs with residual temperature is compressed on treatment areas covered with a waterproof towel and a disposable treatment towel for 10 to 15 minutes to further exert efficacy（Fig. 6-9）.

⑥熨毕。用纱布轻拭治疗部位水迹，立即给患者覆盖被子以保暖（图 6-10）。

⑥ Finishing ironing. The water on treatment areas is lightly cleaned with gauzes and the patient is immediately covered with a blanket to keep him/her warm（Fig. 6-10）.

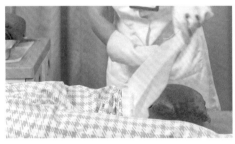
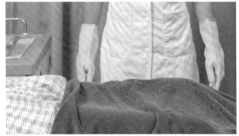

图 6-9 敷熨

Fig. 6-9　Ironing with the way of compressing

图 6-10 熨毕

Fig. 6-10　Finishing ironing

（5）整理患者衣物及操作物品。

（5）The doctor tidies up the patient's clothing and used materials.

（6）交代患者治疗后注意事项等。

（6）The doctor informs the patient of precautions after treatment.

（7）洗手并记录治疗情况。

（7）The doctor washes hands and makes a record about treatment.

六、疗程
Ⅵ　Course of treatment

每次每个部位 20 ～ 30 分钟，依病情而定。一般每天 1 次，5 ～ 15 天为 1 个疗程。

It takes 20 to 30 minutes for a treatment area each time according to the patient's disease condition. In general，once a day，5 to 15 days as a course of treatment.

七、注意事项
Ⅶ　Notes

（1）患者过度疲劳、过度饥饿、过度饱或精神高度紧张时不能操作。暴露治疗部位时，应注意保护患者隐私及保暖。

（1）It is prohibited for patients who suffer from excessive fatigue，excessive hunger，overeating or high mental stress. When treatment areas are exposed，the doctor should protect the patient's privacy and keep the patient warm.

（2）治疗过程中随时观察患者局部皮肤及病情，随时询问患者耐受程度。

（2）During this process，the doctor should observe the patient's skin and condition as well as ask the patient's tolerance to this therapy at any time.

（3）嘱患者皮肤轻微发红为正常现象，如有疼痛、起水疱要及时告知医护人员予以处理。

（3）Tell the patient that there will be slight redness on the skin of treatment areas. If there is pain or blisters，the patient should tell the medical staff timely.

（4）烫熨后 4 ～ 6 小时内不得洗澡，不吹冷风，注意保暖；忌食寒性、热性、酸辣刺激之品。

（4）Do not take a bath within 4 to 6 hours after ironing and keep warm. Foods that are cold，spicy，and sour should be avoided.

八、意外情况及处理
VIII　Accidents and handling methods

如有烫伤，用生理盐水清洁创面并浸润无菌纱布湿敷创面直至疼痛明显减轻或消失后，外涂烧伤膏。如起小水疱，皮肤可自行吸收，保持局部干燥及水疱皮肤的完整性即可；如水疱较大，可用无菌针头将水疱戳破，放出疱内渗液，每日用碘伏消毒，外涂烧伤膏，保持局部干燥及清洁，预防感染。

For scalds，the surface of the wound should be cleaned with physiological saline and compressed by wet sterile gauzes until the pain is greatly relieved or disappears，and then applied burn ointment. For small blisters，the skin will absorb the blisters fluid if the skin over the blisters is not open and kept dry. For large blisters，a sterile needle can be used to puncture them to release the fluid. The patient should disinfect it with iodophor，apply burn ointment to it，and keep the skin dry and clean to prevent infection.

【附注】
【Notes】

烫熨壮医方
Traditional Zhuang Medicine Prescription about Ironing

将柑叶 100 g、大罗伞 100 g、两面针 50 g、五色梅 50 g、土荆芥 50 g、柚叶 50 g 等壮药用 45 度米酒浸泡，放在缸内密封泡制。

Ganye（Folium Citri Reticulatae）100 g，Daluosan（Radix Ardisiae Crenatae）100 g，Liangmianzhen（Radix zanthoxyli）50 g，Wusemei（Folium Lantanae Camarae）50 g，Tujingjie（Herba Chenopodii Ambrosiodis）50 g，Youye（Folium Citri Grandis）50 g and other Zhuang herbs are put into a jar with rice wine（45% vol）. Then，the jar is sealed.

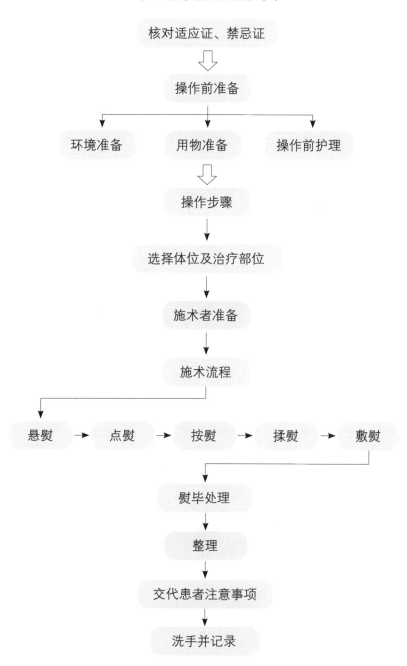

壮医熨烫疗法流程图

The Flow Chart about Zhuang Medicine Ironing Therapy

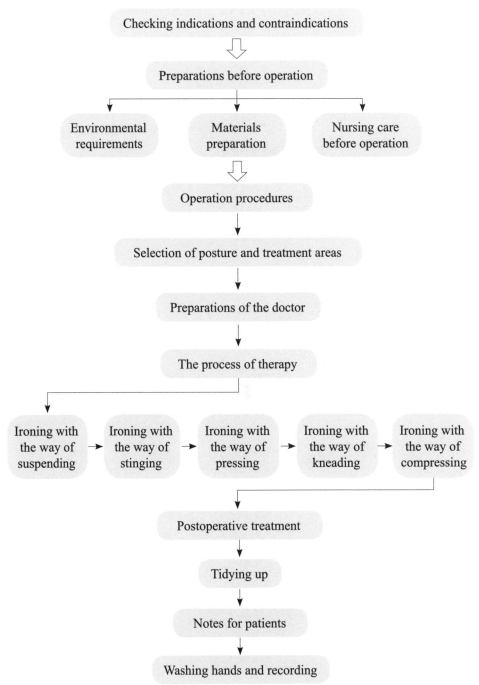

第七章　壮医药物竹罐疗法
Chapter 7　Zhuang Medicine Bamboo Cupping Therapy

壮医药物竹罐疗法是将特制的竹罐放入煮沸的壮药药液中加热，再将竹罐趁热吸附于治疗部位上，以治疗疾病的一种方法。

Zhuang medicine bamboo cupping therapy refers to a therapeutic method of putting special bamboo cups into the boiling Zhuang medicinal solution, then placing the bamboo cups on treatment areas to treat diseases.

一、主要功效
Ⅰ　Main effects

祛风、湿、痧、瘴、寒、痰、瘀等毒，消肿，散结，通痹，止痛，通调三道两路，调节气血平衡。

To dispel wind, dampness, pathogen, miasma, cold, phlegm and blood stasis. To eliminate swelling, stagnation, arthralgia spasm and pain. To regulate three passages and two pathways and the balance between qi and blood.

二、适应证
Ⅱ　Indications

各科疾病均可使用本疗法治疗，主要用于寒毒、瘀毒所致的病证，常见适应证有发旺（痹病）、贫痧（痧症）、核尹（腰痛）、活邀尹（颈椎病）、麻抹（麻木）、麻邦（中风）、骆扔（骨折愈后瘀积）、林得叮相（跌打损伤）、巧尹（头痛）、㾟呗嘟（带状疱疹、带状疱疹后遗神经痛）等。

This therapy can be used to treat common diseases, mainly diseases caused by cold and blood stasis. Its common indications include Fawang（arthralgia disease）, Pinsha（acute filthy disease）, Heyin（low back pain）, Huoyaoyin （cervical spondylosis）, Mamo（numbness）, Mabang（stroke）, Luoreng（healing stasis after fracture）, Lindedingxiang（traumatic injury）, Qiaoyin（headache）, Benbeilang（shingles, postherpetic neuralgia）, etc.

三、禁忌证
Ⅲ　Contraindications

（1）自发出血性疾病患者、有出血倾向或凝血功能障碍者禁用。

（1）It is prohibited for patients who have spontaneous hemorrhagic diseases and coagulation disorders.

（2）严重心脑血管疾病患者、血糖控制不佳者、精神病患者、身体极度虚弱消瘦或皮肤没有弹性者禁用。

（2）It is prohibited for patients who have severe cardiovascular and cerebrovascular diseases, poor glycemic control, psychosis, or an extremely weak constitution or poor skin elasticity.

（3）过度疲劳、过度饥饿、过度饱或精神高度紧张的患者禁用。

（3）It is prohibited for patients who suffer from excessive fatigue, excessive hunger, overeating or high mental stress.

（4）局部皮肤有破溃、疤痕、高度水肿处及体表大血管处禁用。

（4）It is prohibited for patients who suffer from skin ulcers, scars or severe edema as well as superficial large vessels.

（5）孕妇禁用。

（5）It is prohibited for pregnant women.

四、操作前准备
Ⅳ　Preparations before operation

（1）环境要求。治疗室内清洁，安静，光线明亮，温度适宜，避免患者吹风受凉。

（1）Environmental requirements. The treatment room should be clean，quiet，well-lit. Besides，keep the treatment room at an ideal temperature to prevent the patient from catching a cold.

（2）用物准备。

（2）Materials preparation.

①竹罐（图 7-1）、电磁炉、不锈钢锅（图 7-2）或其他锅具、消毒毛巾、长镊子（图 7-3）、一次性注射针头、一次性无菌手套、复合碘皮肤消毒液、医用棉签、无菌纱布、医用干棉球。

①Bamboo cups（Fig. 7-1），an induction cooker，a stainless steel pot（Fig. 7-2）or other pots，disinfected towels，long forceps（Fig. 7-3），disposable injection needles，disposable sterile gloves，compound iodine skin disinfectant，medical cotton swabs，sterile gauzes，medical dry cotton balls.

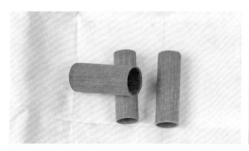

图 7-1 竹罐
Fig. 7-1 Bamboo cups

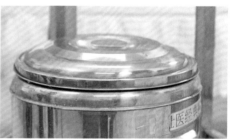

图 7-2 不锈钢锅
Fig. 7-2 A stainless steel pot

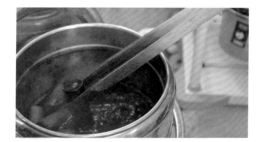

图 7-3 长镊子
Fig. 7-3 Long forceps

②药物。根据病证选择相应的壮药。

② Zhuang medicinal materials. The appropriate Zhuang medicinal materials are selected according to the disease pattern.

③药液。将药物装入布袋（图 7-4），加水浸泡至少 30 分钟，然后放入锅具内加热煮沸用于浸煮竹罐（图 7-5）。

③ Medicinal solution. These herbs are put into a bag（Fig. 7-4）and soaked in water for at least 30 minutes, and then placed in a pot to be boiled for steeping bamboo cups（Fig. 7-5）.

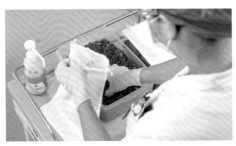
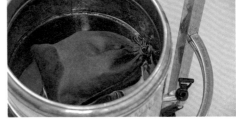

图 7-4　装药　　　　　　　　　　　图 7-5　放药袋入水中
Fig. 7-4　Putting herbs into a bag　　Fig. 7-5　Putting the bag filled with herbs into water

（3）操作前护理。核对患者信息及治疗方案等，说明治疗的意义和注意事项，取得患者同意；对患者进行精神安慰与鼓励，消除患者的紧张、恐惧情绪，使患者能积极主动配合操作。

（3）Nursing care before operation. The nurse should check the patient's information and treatment plan and explain the significance and notices of the treatment to obtain the patient's consent. Besides, the nurse should encourage the patient to overcome his/her nervousness and fear and enable the patient to cooperate with the doctor for a better operation.

五、操作步骤
V　Operation procedures

（1）体位选择。根据患者病情确定体位，常取坐位、俯卧位、仰卧位、侧卧位等，以患者舒适及便于施术者操作为宜，避免用强迫体位。

（1）Posture selection. Based on the state of the illness, the posture is selected. Sitting position，prone position，dorsal position or lateral recumbent position is often selected to provide convenience for the patient and the doctor. The compulsive position should be avoided.

（2）部位选择。根据病证选取适当的治疗部位或穴位，常选局部阿是穴为主，可配合邻近部位取穴。每次治疗部位不超过4个。

（2）Position selection. The appropriate treatment areas and acupoints are selected according to the disease pattern. Ashi acupoint is often selected，combined with acupoints near the adjacent parts. The number of treatment areas should not exceed 4.

（3）洗手，戴医用外科口罩、医用帽子和一次性无菌手套。

（3）The doctor should wash hands，wear a surgical mask，a medical cap and disposable sterile gloves.

（4）施术流程。

（4）Operation procedures.

①煮罐。将竹罐投入药液中，煮沸5分钟后备用（图7-6）。

① Cup boiling. The bamboo cups are put into the solution and boiled for 5 minutes（Fig. 7-6）.

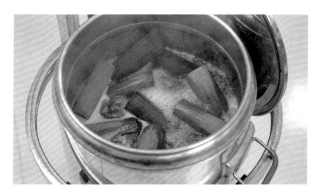

图 7-6　浸煮竹罐

Fig. 7-6　Cup boiling

②拔罐。根据拔罐部位选定大小合适的竹罐。夹取竹罐（图7-7），用折叠的消毒毛巾捂一下罐口（图7-8），以便吸去罐内的药液，降低罐口的温度和保持罐内的热气，然后迅速扣拔于选定的部位或穴位上（图7-9）。根据病

情及治疗部位确定拔罐数量，5～10分钟后，按压罐边使空气进入并取下竹罐（图7-10）。

② Cupping. The proper bamboo cups are selected according to treatment areas and the bamboo cups are taken out（Fig. 7-7）. Then，the mouth of the cup is covered with a folded disinfected towel（Fig. 7-8）in order to clean the medicinal solution in the cup，lower the temperature of the mouth of the cup and keep the temperature in the cup，and then quickly put it on the selected parts or acupoints（Fig. 7-9）. The number of cupping is determined according to the disease condition and treatment area. After 5 to 10 minutes，the skin along the edge of cup is pressed to let the air in，then，bamboo cups are removed（Fig. 7-10）.

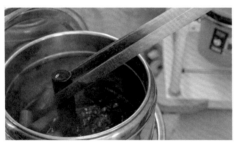

图7-7　夹取竹罐

Fig. 7-7　Taking bamboo cups out

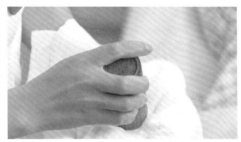

图7-8　捂住罐口

Fig. 7-8　Covering the mouth of the cup

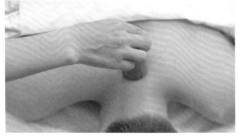

图7-9　扣拔竹罐

Fig. 7-9　Cupping

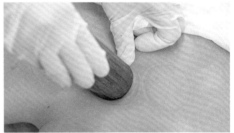

图7-10　取下竹罐

Fig. 7-10　Removal of bamboo cups

③竹罐热熨。再次从锅中夹出竹罐（图7-7），用折叠的消毒毛巾捂一下罐口（图7-8），以便吸去罐内的药液，待热度合适后滚动竹罐热熨于治疗部位（图7-11）。热熨约5分钟。

③ Ironing the skin with bamboo cups. The bamboo cups are taken out from the pot（Fig. 7-7）, then, the mouth of the cup is covered with a folded disinfected towel（Fig. 7-8）to clean the medicinal solution in the cup. Then, the doctor rolls the warm cup to iron treatment areas（Fig. 7-11）. It lasts for about 5 minutes.

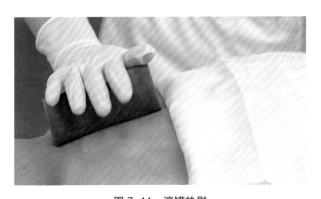

图 7-11　滚罐热熨

Fig. 7-11　Rolling the warm cup to iron

一般拔罐过程到此即可结束。但如为急性病患者、体质较好的慢性病患者或拔罐部位瘀血较重者，暂不宜做热熨，可继续做壮医刺血和再次拔罐，具体如下。

In general, this is the whole cupping process. But for patients who have acute diseases, chronic diseases but good constitution or severe blood stasis, ironing is not advisable. The doctor can perform blood-letting therapy and cupping again to these patients. The process is as follows.

④刺血。根据患者病情选择相应罐印部位或穴位进行壮医刺血。常规消毒皮肤，用一次性注射针头在罐印部位或穴位皮肤上迅速浅刺1～3针（图7-12），以局部少量渗血为度。

④ Blood-letting. The acupoints of blood-letting are determined according to the patient's disease condition and location. Firstly, the skin is disinfected. Then, the doctor quickly performs 1 to 3 blood-letting on treatment areas with a disposable injection needle（Fig. 7-12）. Small amount of blood oozing is proper.

⑤再次拔罐。另取煮热的竹罐在刺血部位再次拔罐（图7-13），5～10分钟后取下竹罐，用消毒干棉球擦净针刺部位的血迹，常规消毒皮肤。

⑤ Cupping again. Treatment areas can be performed cupping again with warm bamboo cups（Fig. 7-13）for 5 ～ 10 minutes. Then the bamboo cups are removed，and the blood on treatment areas are cleaned with disinfected cotton balls.

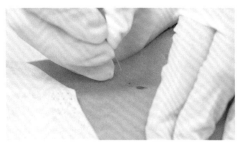

图 7-12　刺血

Fig.7 -12　Blood-letting

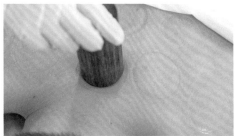

图 7-13　再次放罐

Fig.7 -13　Cupping again

（5）整理患者衣物及操作物品。

（5）The doctor tidies up the patient's clothing and used materials.

（6）交代患者治疗后注意事项等。

（6）The doctor informs the patient of precautions after treatment.

（7）洗手并记录治疗情况。

（7）The doctor washes hands and makes a record about treatment.

六、疗程
Ⅵ　Course of treatment

每次治疗 40 ～ 50 分钟，2 ～ 3 天 1 次，5 ～ 7 次为 1 个疗程。

Each treatment lasts 40 to 50 minutes，once every 2 to 3 days，5 ～ 7 times as a course of treatment.

七、注意事项
Ⅶ　Notes

（1）患者过度疲劳、过度饥饿、过度饱或精神高度紧张时不能操作。暴露治疗部位时，应注意保护患者隐私及保暖。

（1）It is prohibited for patients who suffer from excessive fatigue, excessive hunger, overeating or high mental stress. When treatment areas are exposed, the doctor should protect the patient's privacy and keep the patient warm.

（2）治疗过程中随时观察患者局部皮肤及病情，随时询问患者耐受程度。

（2）During this process, the doctor should observe the patient's skin and condition as well as ask the patient's tolerance to this therapy at any time.

（3）拔罐前尽量甩干水珠以免烫伤患者皮肤。

（3）Try to remove the water on the cups as much as possible before cupping to avoid scalding the patient's skin.

（4）嘱患者拔罐过程中不可随便移动体位，以免引起疼痛或竹罐脱落。

（4）Tell the patient not to change the posture during the cupping process to avoid pain or cup shedding.

（5）选择肌肉丰厚、皮下组织松弛及毛发少的部位为宜，多毛部位需剃毛。

（5）The position with thick muscles, loose subcutaneous tissue and little hair should be selected and the hair on the hairy areas needs to be shaved.

（6）取罐时动作要轻柔，按压罐边使空气进入即可取下，不能硬拉竹罐。

（6）The cup should be removed gently. The doctor should press the skin along the edge of the cup to let the air in and remove it.

（7）施术后可予患者饮温开水。

（7）After the operation, the patient can drink some warm water.

（8）嘱患者拔罐后当天避免接触冷水，注意保暖。

（8）Tell the patient to avoid being exposed to cold water after cupping and keep warm on that day.

（9）使用过的竹罐、毛巾送消毒供应中心统一消毒。

（9）Used bamboo cups and towels should be sent to central sterile supply department to be disinfected.

八、意外情况及处理
VIII Accidents and handling methods

（1）晕罐。立即停止拔罐，让患者头低位平卧，亦可加服少量糖水；若出现严重至昏迷不醒者，立即行急救处理。

（1）Fainting. The cupping should be stopped immediately. Help the patient lie flat with head-down tilt and drink a small amount of sugar water. If the patient is unconscious，an emergency treatment should be performed immediately.

（2）烫伤、起水疱。如有烫伤，用生理盐水清洁创面并浸润无菌纱布湿敷创面直至疼痛明显减轻或消失后，外涂烧伤膏。如起小水疱，皮肤可自行吸收，保持局部干燥及水疱皮肤的完整性即可；如水疱较大，可用无菌针头将水疱戳破，放出疱内渗液，每日用碘伏消毒，外涂烧伤膏，保持局部干燥及清洁，预防感染。

（2）Scalds and blisters. For scalds，the surface of the wound should be cleaned with physiological saline and compressed by wet sterile gauzes until the pain is greatly relieved or disappears，and then applied burn ointment. For small blisters，the skin will absorb the blisters fluid if the skin over the blisters is not open and kept dry. For large blisters，a sterile needle can be used to puncture them to release the fluid. The patient should disinfect it with iodophor，apply burn ointment to it，and keep the skin dry and clean every day to prevent infection.

【附注】
【Notes】

壮医药物竹罐疗法各治疗部位及拔罐数量

治疗部位	拔罐数量
颈部（包括上背、颈）	12 罐
背部	20 罐
腰部	20 罐
单侧肩关节（包括肩周、肩胛区）	16 罐
单侧肘关节（包括肘、上臂、前臂）	10 罐
单侧腕关节（包括腕、手背、前臂）	6 罐
双侧臀部	16 罐
单侧膝关节	10 罐
单侧踝关节	8 罐
单侧上肢	12 罐
单侧下肢	16 罐

The Number of Bamboo Cups Used for Each Part of Zhuang Medicine Bamboo Cupping Therapy

Body parts	Number of cups
Neck（including upper back and neck）	12 cups
Back	20 cups
Waist	20 cups
Unilateral shoulder joint（including scapula and scapular region）	16 cups
Unilateral elbow joint（including elbow，upper arm，forearm）	10 cups
Unilateral wrist joint（including wrist，back of hand，forearm）	6 cups
Bilateral buttocks	16 cups
Unilateral knee joint	10 cups
Unilateral ankle joint	8 cups
Unilateral upper limb	12 cups
Unilateral lower limb	16 cups

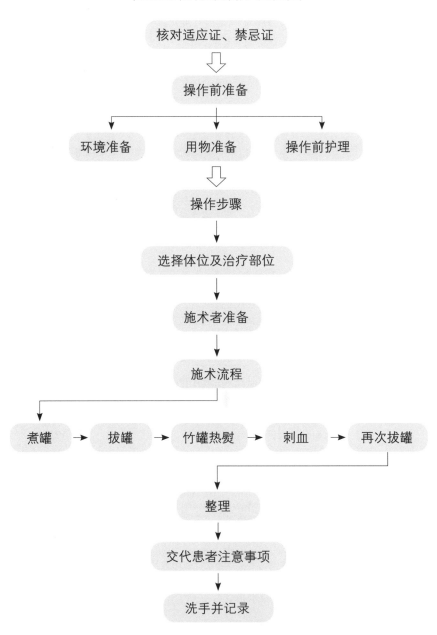

壮医药物竹罐治疗流程图

核对适应证、禁忌证

操作前准备

环境准备　　用物准备　　操作前护理

操作步骤

选择体位及治疗部位

施术者准备

施术流程

煮罐　→　拔罐　→　竹罐热熨　→　刺血　→　再次拔罐

整理

交代患者注意事项

洗手并记录

The Flow Chart about Zhuang Medicine Bamboo Cupping Therapy

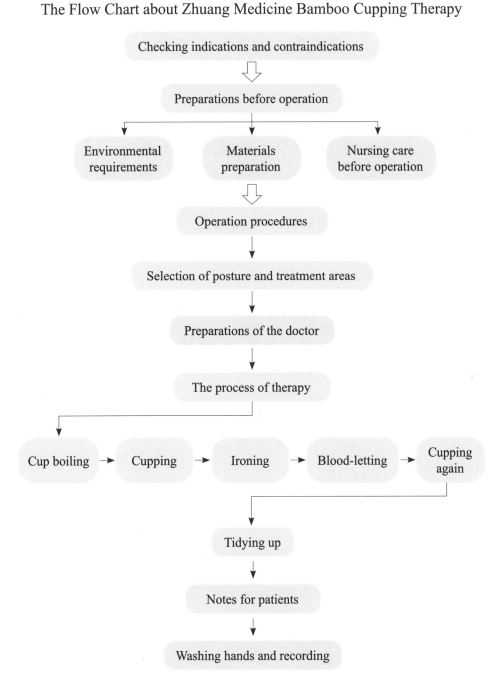

第八章　壮医刺血疗法
Chapter 8　Zhuang Medicine Pricking Blood Therapy

壮医刺血疗法是用针具刺入人体的穴位、病灶、病理反应点和浅表血络，通过挤压、拔罐等放出适量血液，以治疗疾病的一种方法。

Zhuang medicine pricking blood therapy is a therapeutic method of pricking a certain acupoint, lesions, positive reaction points, and superficial venules and applying squeezing or cupping to make the blood out.

一、主要功效
Ⅰ　Main effects

祛风、湿、痧、瘴、热、痰、瘀等毒，消肿，散结，止痛，通调三道两路，调节气血平衡。

To dispel wind, dampness, pathogen, miasma, fever, phlegm and blood stasis. To eliminate swelling, stagnation, and pain. To regulate three passages and two pathways and the balance between qi and blood.

二、适应证
Ⅱ　Indications

内科、外科、妇科、皮肤科等常见病、多发病均可使用本疗法治疗，常见适应证有贫痧（痧症）、发旺（痹病）、核嘎尹（腰腿痛）、活邀尹（颈椎病）、旁巴尹（肩周炎）、骆芡（骨性关节炎）、麻抹（麻木）、甫裆呷（半身不遂）、林得叮相（跌打损伤）、年闹诺（失眠）、巧尹（头痛）、嗓呗啷（带状疱疹、带状疱疹后遗神经痛）、能啥累（瘙痒、湿疹）、叻仇（痤疮）等。

This therapy can be used to treat the common diseases and frequently-occurring diseases of internal medicine，surgery，gynecology，dermatology，etc. Its common indications include Pinsha（acute filthy disease），Fawang（arthralgia disease），Hegayin（lumbocrural pain），Huoyaoyin（cervical spondylosis），Pangbayin（scapulohumeral periarthritis），Luoqian（osteoarthritis），Mamo（numbness），Bengdangxia（hemiplegia），Lindedingxiang（traumatic injury），Niannaonuo（insomnia），Qiaoyin（headache），Benbeilang（shingles，postherpetic neuralgia），Nenghanlei（pruritus，eczema），Lechou（acne），etc.

三、禁忌证
Ⅲ Contraindications

（1）自发出血性疾病患者、凝血功能障碍者禁用。

（1）It is prohibited for patients who have spontaneous hemorrhagic diseases and coagulation disorders.

（2）严重心脑血管疾病患者、血糖控制不佳者、精神病患者、身体极度消瘦虚弱者等禁用。

（2）It is prohibited for patients who have severe cardiovascular and cerebrovascular diseases，poor glycemic control，psychosis，or an extremely weak constitution.

（3）局部皮肤有破溃、疤痕、高度水肿处及浅表大血管处禁用。

（3）It is prohibited for patients who have skin ulcers，scars，severe edema，and superficial large vessels.

（4）过度疲劳、过度饥饿、过度饱或精神高度紧张的患者禁用。

（4）It is prohibited for patients who suffer from excessive fatigue，excessive hunger，overeating or high mental stress.

（5）孕妇禁用。

（5）It is prohibited for pregnant women.

四、操作前准备

Ⅳ Preparations before operation

（1）环境要求。治疗室内清洁，安静，光线明亮，温度适宜，避免患者吹风受凉。

（1）Environmental requirements. The treatment room should be clean, quiet, well-lit. Besides, keep the treatment room at an ideal temperature to prevent the patient from catching a cold.

（2）用物准备。一次性三棱针或注射器针头（图8-1）、一次性无菌手套、复合碘皮肤消毒液、75%酒精、医用棉签或干棉球、无菌纱布或创可贴、胶布。

（2）Materials preparation. Disposable three-edged needles or syringe needles （Fig. 8-1）, disposable sterile gloves, compound iodine skin disinfectant, 75% alcohol, medical cotton swabs or dry cotton balls, sterile gauzes or Band-Aid, adhesive plaster.

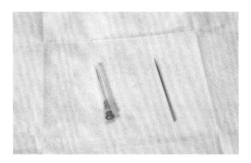

图 8-1　一次性三棱针（右）和注射器针头（左）

Fig. 8-1　A disposable three-edged needle（right）and a syringe needle（left）

（3）操作前护理。核对患者信息及治疗方案等，说明治疗的意义和注意事项，取得患者同意；对患者进行精神安慰与鼓励，消除患者的紧张、恐惧情绪，使患者能积极主动配合操作。

（3）Nursing care before operation. The nurse should check the patient's information and treatment plan and explain the significance and notices of the treatment to obtain the patient's consent. Besides, the nurse should encourage the patient to overcome his/her nervousness and fear and enable the patient to cooperate with the doctor for a better operation.

五、操作步骤
V　Operation procedures

（1）体位选择。根据患者病情确定体位，常取坐位、俯卧位、仰卧位、侧卧位等，以患者舒适及便于施术者操作为宜，避免用强迫体位。

（1）Posture selection. Based on the state of the illness，the posture is selected. Sitting position，prone position，dorsal position，or lateral recumbent position is often selected to provide convenience for the patient and the doctor. The compulsive position should be avoided.

（2）定位。根据病证选取适当的治疗部位。

（2）Location selection. According to the disease patterns，the corresponding treatment area is selected.

（3）洗手，戴医用外科口罩、医用帽子和一次性无菌手套。

（3）The doctor should wash hands，then wear a surgical mask，a medical cap and disposable sterile gloves.

（4）消毒。

（4）Disinfection.

①针具。选择一次性三棱针或注射器针头。

① Needles. A disposable three-edged needle or a syringe needle is selected.

②部位。常规消毒施术部位皮肤，消毒范围的直径大于施术部位 5 cm。

② Parts. The related skin is disinfected，and the diameter of the disinfection areas is larger than that of treatment areas（exceeding 5 cm）.

（5）施术流程。

（5）Operation procedures.

①持针。右手拇指、食指二指持针（图 8-2），中指抵住针体，露出针尖 1～2 cm（图 8-3），左手捏住或夹持刺血部位皮肤。

① Needle holding. The thumb and index finger of the right hand hold the needle（Fig. 8-2），then，the middle finger keeps the needle body and 1 to 2 cm of the needle tip is exposed（Fig. 8-3）, and then the skin of treatment part is pinched by the left hand.

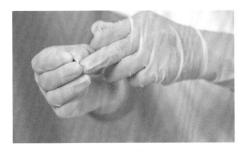

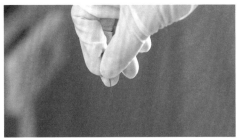

图 8-2 持针手势
Fig. 8-2 Gesture of needle holding

图 8-3 进针手势
Fig. 8-3 Gesture of needle inserting

②进针。右手持针迅速浅刺治疗部位（图 8-4），进针深度为 0.1 ~ 0.3 cm，左手挤按针孔使之出血（图 8-5）。

② Needle inserting. The needle is held to prick the treatment part quickly with the right hand（Fig. 8-4）. The depth of needle insertion is 0.1 to 0.3 cm. The pinhole is pressed by the left hand to cause bleeding（Fig. 8-5）.

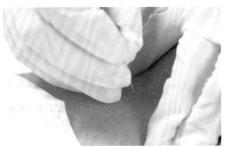

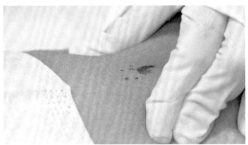

图 8-4 浅刺
Fig. 8-4 Shallow pricking

图 8-5 刺血后
Fig. 8-5 After pricking

③根据患者病情加用拔罐以增加出血量（图 8-6）。

③ According to the patient's disease condition，cupping is added to increase the amount of bleeding（Fig. 8-6）.

④用无菌纱布擦拭所拔部位流出的瘀血，常规消毒治疗部位的皮肤。

④ The ecchymosis at the treatment part is wiped with sterile gauzes and the skin of treatment part is routinely disinfected.

（6）施术后处理。用过的针具置于利器盒中销毁处理。

（6）Postoperative treatment. The used needles should be put in a sharps box.

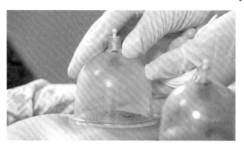

图 8-6 拔罐

Fig. 8-6 Cupping

（7）整理患者衣物及操作物品。

（7）The doctor tidies up the patient's clothing and used materials.

（8）交代患者治疗后注意事项等。

（8）The doctor informs the patient of precautions after treatment.

（9）洗手并记录治疗情况。

（9）The doctor washes hands and makes a record about treatment.

六、疗程
Ⅵ Course of treatment

急性病证 1 ～ 2 天 1 次，慢性病证 3 ～ 5 天 1 次，5 次为 1 个疗程。

For acute disease，once every 1 to 2 days；for chronic disease，once every 3 to 5 days，5 times as a course of treatment.

七、注意事项
Ⅶ Notes

（1）患者过于疲劳、过于饥饿、过于饱或精神高度紧张时不能操作。暴露治疗部位时，应注意保护患者隐私及保暖。

（1）It is prohibited for patients who suffer from excessive fatigue，excessive hunger, overeating or high mental stress. When treated areas are exposed, the doctor should protect the patient's privacy and keep the patient warm.

（2）治疗过程中随时观察局部皮肤及病情，随时询问患者的耐受程度。

（2）During this process, the doctor should observe the patient's skin and condition as well as ask the patient's tolerance to this therapy at any time.

（3）点刺时，手法宜轻、浅、快。

（3）When pricking, the doctor should adopt this manipulation technique that is gentle, shallow, and fast.

（4）注意切勿刺伤深部大动脉。

（4）Do not prick the aorta.

（5）操作过程中应遵守无菌操作规则，防止感染。

（5）Aseptic operation should be obeyed during treatment to prevent infection.

（6）治疗后避免患者立即起身离开，为其安排舒适体位，嘱其休息5～10分钟后方可活动。

（6）Prevent the patient from getting up and leaving immediately after treatment. Let the patient take a comfortable posture and rest for 5 to 10 minutes.

（7）操作后必须交代患者，若施术部位有瘙痒，属正常的治疗反应，避免用手抓破，以免引起感染。保持施术部位皮肤清洁干燥，6小时内不宜洗澡。

（7）After the operation, the patient should be instructed that itching on treatment areas is a normal treatment reaction and do not scratch this part. Keep the skin of treatment part clean and dry, do not take a bath within 6 hours.

八、意外情况及处理

Ⅷ　Accidents and handling methods

（1）晕针、晕罐。如患者治疗过程中出现气短、面色苍白、出冷汗等晕针现象，立即让患者头低位平卧10分钟左右，亦可加服少量糖水；若出现严重至昏迷不醒者，立即行急救处理。

（1）Fainting. If the patient develops shortness of breath, pale complexion and cold sweat during treatment, this operation should be stopped immediately, and help the patient lie flat with head-down tilt for about 10 minutes and drink a small amount of sugar water. If the patient is unconscious，an emergency treatment should be performed immediately.

（2）血肿。用消毒干棉球按压血肿部位针孔 3 ～ 5 分钟，防止血肿变大。出血量较大的血肿可加以冷敷，以促进凝血，48 小时后可行热敷促进血肿吸收。

（2）Hematoma. The pinhole of the hematoma part should be pressed with a disinfected dry cotton ball for 3 to 5 minutes to avoid larger hematoma. The hematoma with a large amount of bleeding should be treated with cold compressing firstly to promote coagulation and the hot compressing after 48 hours to promote the absorption of hematoma.

【附注】
【Notes】

壮医刺血疗法出血量估算
Estimation of the Amount of Bleeding of Zhuang Medicine Pricking Blood Therapy

微量：出血量≤ 1.0 mL。

Slight amount：the amount of bleeding ≤ 1.0 mL.

少量：出血量在 1.1 ～ 5.0 mL。

Small amount：the amount of bleeding is 1.1 to 5.0 mL.

中等量：出血量在 5.1 ～ 10.0 mL。

Medium amount：the amount of bleeding is 5.1 to 10.0 mL.

大量：出血量＞ 10.0 mL。

Large amount：the amount of bleeding ＞ 10.0 mL.

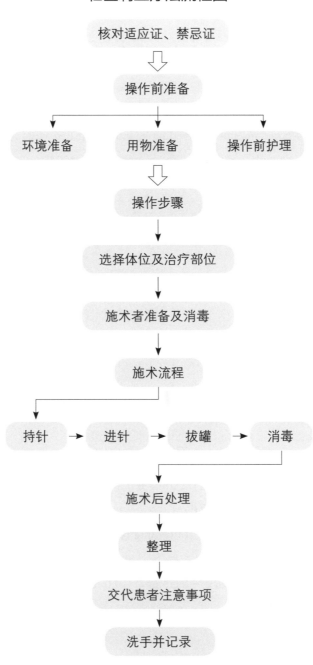

壮医刺血疗法流程图

The Flow Chart about Zhuang Medicine Pricking Blood Therapy

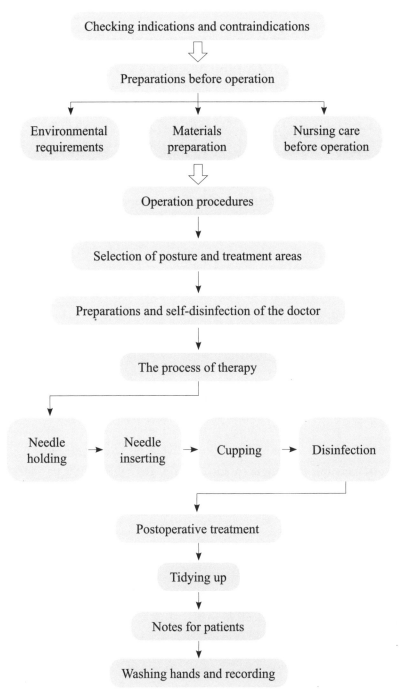

第九章　壮医火攻疗法
Chapter 9　Zhuang Medicine Fire Therapy

壮医火攻疗法是用双层牛皮纸包裹熄灭明火后的药枝或药藤，或点燃药枝或药藤待明火熄灭后，直接隔着双层牛皮纸熨灸于患者体表部位或穴位，以治疗疾病的一种方法。

Zhuang medicine fire therapy refers to a therapeutic method of burning the prepared medicinal twigs or medicinal vines till the naked flame disappears and then wrapping it with kraft paper which is put upon the affected areas or acupoints to treat the disease.

一、主要功效
I　Main effects

祛风、湿、寒、痰、瘀等毒，消肿，散结，通痹，止痛，通调三道两路，调节气血平衡。

To dispel wind, dampness, cold, phlegm and blood stasis. To eliminate swelling, stagnation, arthralgia spasm and pain. To regulate three passages and two pathways and the balance between qi and blood.

二、适应证
II　Indications

内科、外科、妇科、儿科等常见病、多发病均可使用本疗法治疗，常见适应证有巧尹（头痛）、发旺（痹病）、核嘎尹（腰腿痛）、活邀尹（颈椎病）、旁巴尹（肩周炎）、滚克（类风湿关节炎）、麻抹（麻木）、扭相（软组织挫伤）、腊胴尹（腹痛）、白冻（腹泻）、京尹（痛经）、嘻缶（乳腺增生）等。

This therapy can be used to treat the common diseases and frequently-occurring diseases of internal medicine，surgery，gynecology，pediatrics，etc. Its common indications include Qiaoyin（headache），Fawang（arthralgia disease），Hegayin（lumbocrural pain），Huoyaoyin（cervical spondylosis），Pangbayin（scapulohumeral periarthritis），Gunke（rheumatoid arthritis），Mamo（numbness），Niuxiang（soft tissue contusion），Ladongyin（abdominal pain），Baidong（diarrhea），Jingyin（dysmenorrhea），Xifou（hyperplasia of mammary glands），etc.

三、禁忌证
Ⅲ　Contraindications

（1）辨证为阳证患者禁用。

（1）It is prohibited for patients with Yang syndrome.

（2）发热（体温≥37.3 ℃）、脉搏≥90 次 / 分患者禁用。

（2）It is prohibited for patients with fever（body temperature ≥ 37.3 ℃）or pulse rate ≥ 90 beats/min.

（3）开放性创口、感染性病灶、疤痕、高度水肿处、黏膜及浅表大血管处禁用。

（3）It is prohibited for treatment areas with open wounds，infectious lesions，scars and severe edema. Besides，it is prohibited for mucosa and superficial large vessels.

（4）过度疲劳、过度饥饿、过度饱或精神高度紧张的患者禁用。

（4）It is prohibited for patients who suffer from excessive fatigue，excessive hunger，overeating or high mental stress.

（5）严重心脑血管疾病患者、血糖控制不佳者、精神病患者、身体极度消瘦虚弱者等禁用。

（5）It is prohibited for patients who have severe cardiovascular and cerebrovascular diseases，poor glycemic control，psychosis，or an extremely weak constitution.

四、操作前准备

IV　Preparations before operation

（1）环境要求。治疗室内清洁，安静，光线明亮，温度适宜，避免患者吹风受凉。

（1）Environmental requirements. The treatment room should be clean, quiet, well-lit. Besides, keep the treatment room at an ideal temperature to prevent the patient from catching a cold.

（2）用物准备。

（2）Materials preparation.

①加工炮制过的药枝或药藤（每段长 15 ～ 20 cm，图 9-1）。

① Processed medicinal twigs or medicinal vines（each with the length of 15 to 20 cm，Fig. 9-1）.

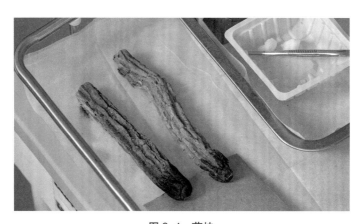

图 9-1　药枝
Fig. 9-1　Medicinal twigs

②牛皮纸、酒精灯、打火机、纱布、灭火盒、一次性无菌手套。

② Kraft paper，an alcohol lamp，a lighter，gauzes，a fire extinguisher box，disposable sterile gloves.

（3）操作前护理。核对患者信息及治疗方案等，说明治疗的意义和注意事项，取得患者同意；对患者进行精神安慰与鼓励，消除患者的紧张、恐惧情绪，使患者能积极主动配合操作。

（3）Nursing care before operation. The nurse should check the patient's information and treatment plan and explain the significance and notices of the treatment to obtain the patient's consent. Besides, the nurse should encourage the patient to overcome his/her nervousness and fear and enable the patient to cooperate with the doctor for a better operation.

五、操作步骤
V　Operation procedures

（1）体位选择。根据患者病情确定体位，常取坐位、俯卧位、仰卧位、侧卧位等，以患者舒适及便于施术者操作为宜，避免用强迫体位。

（1）Posture selection. Based on the state of the illness, the posture is determined. Sitting position, prone position, dorsal position, or lateral recumbent position is often selected to provide convenience for the patient and the doctor. The compulsive position should be avoided.

（2）定位。根据病证选取相应治疗部位。

（2）Location selection. According to the disease patterns, the corresponding treatment area is selected.

（3）洗手，戴医用外科口罩、医用帽子和一次性无菌手套。

（3）The doctor should wash hands, wear a surgical mask, a medical cap and disposable sterile gloves.

（4）清洁。用生理盐水清洁治疗部位的皮肤。

（4）Cleaning. Clean the skin of treatment areas with physiological saline.

（5）施术流程。

（5）Operation procedures.

①选药枝或药藤。选用大小合适、方便操作的药枝或药藤。

① Selecting medicinal twigs or medicinal vines. The medicinal twigs or medicinal vines with appropriate sizes and convenient operation are selected.

②点燃药枝或药藤。将药枝或药藤的一端放在酒精灯上燃烧（图9-2）。

② Igniting the medicinal twig or medicinal vine. One end of the medicinal twig or medicinal vine is burned with an alcohol lamp（Fig. 9-2）.

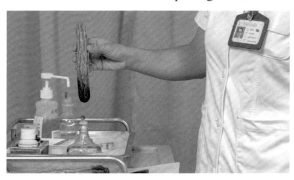

图 9-2　点燃药枝

Fig. 9-2　Igniting the medicinal twig

③包药枝或药藤。待明火熄灭后，用两层牛皮纸将燃着暗火的药枝或药藤（图 9-3）包裹住（图 9-4）。亦可不包药枝或药藤、直接隔着双层牛皮纸熨灸治疗部位。

③ Wrapping the medicinal twig or medicinal vine. After naked flame is extinguished，wrap the medicinal twig or medicinal vine that is with a fire without flames（Fig. 9-3）with two layers of kraft paper（Fig. 9-4）. Or do not wrap the medicinal twig or medicinal vine and directly iron treatment areas with two layers of kraft paper on the skin.

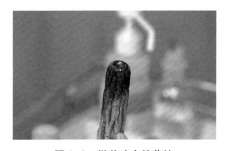

图 9-3　燃着暗火的药枝

Fig. 9-3　The medicinal twig with a fire without flames

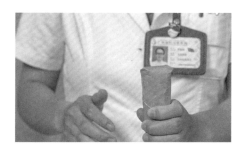

图 9-4　包药枝

Fig. 9-4　Wrapping the medicinal twig

④熨灸。用包裹好的药枝或药藤在患者身上特定部位或穴位熨灸（图 9-5、图 9-6）；或将燃着暗火的药枝或药藤隔着双层牛皮纸直接熨在需熨灸部位上，一上一下熨灸。起初药枝或药藤温度高，熨灸需如鸟啄食样一上一下快速操作，

待温度下降后，熨灸速度可渐慢下来，以患者耐受为标准，以皮肤微微潮红为度（图 9-7）。

④ Ironing. The wrapped medicinal twig or medicinal vine is used to iron on specific parts of the patient's body or acupoints（Fig. 9-5）; or the medicinal twig or medicinal vine with a fire without flames is used to iron on the treatment areas directly with two layers of kraft paper on the skin（Fig. 9-6）. At first, the temperature of the medicinal twig or medicinal vine is high, so the ironing is quickly operated like bird pecking. After the temperature drops, the speed of ironing can gradually slow down. The operation is based on the patient's tolerance and it is better to make the skin slightly flushed（Fig. 9-7）.

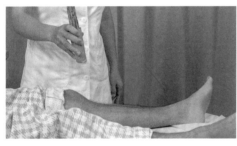

图 9-5　包灸

Fig. 9-5　Ironing with the wrapped medicinal twig or medicinal vine

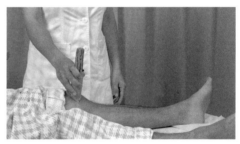

图 9-6　包灸

Fig. 9-6　Ironing with the wrapped medicinal twig or medicinal vine

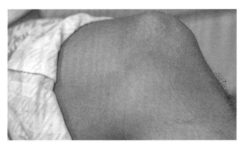

图 9-7　皮肤潮红

Fig. 9-7　Flushed skin

⑤熨毕。用纱布清洁患者局部皮肤。

⑤ Finishing ironing. The patient's local skin is cleaned with gauzes.

（6）施术后处理。将药枝或药藤放入灭火盒内，使之完全熄灭。

（6）Postoperative treatment. The medicinal twig or medicinal vine is put in a fire extinguisher box to completely extinguish the fire.

（7）整理患者衣物及操作物品。

（7）The doctor tidies up the patient's clothing and used materials.

（8）交代患者治疗后注意事项等。

（8）The doctor informs the patient of precautions after treatment.

（9）洗手并记录治疗情况。

（9）The doctor washes hands and makes a record about treatment.

六、疗程
Ⅵ　Course of treatment

一般每天 1 次，病情严重者可每天 2 次，每次可选取不同穴位，10 天为 1 个疗程，每个疗程间隔 1 周。

In general，once a day；severe illness can be twice a day. Different acupoints can be selected every time. 10 days as a course of treatment and its time interval is one week.

七、注意事项
Ⅶ　Notes

（1）患者过度疲劳、过度饥饿、过度饿或精神高度紧张时不能操作。暴露治疗部位时，应注意保护患者隐私及保暖。

（1）It is prohibited for patients who suffer from excessive fatigue，excessive hunger，overeating or high mental stress. When treatment areas are exposed，the doctor should protect the patient's privacy and keep the patient warm.

（2）熨灸过程中如果有热灰脱落，应及时清理，以防烫伤患者皮肤和烧坏衣物。

（2）If there is hot ash during the process of ironing，it should be cleaned timely to avoid scalding the skin and burning clothing.

（3）颜面部、眼周等皮肤细嫩处不宜操作。

（3）Do not operate on face，eyes and other delicate skin.

（4）熨灸过程中要以患者耐受的温度为宜，随时询问患者对熨灸的耐受程度，过热时应当及时撤移药枝或药藤。尤其是半身不遂患者、糖尿病患者及年老体弱者等对温度的感觉反应迟钝，治疗时应注意查看其局部肤色，以局部肤色微微潮红为宜。切忌治疗时过度、过久或用力按压，动作应以轻快为主，以免烫伤患者。

（4）In the process of ironing，it is advisable to ask the patient's tolerance at any time. When overheating，the doctor should promptly remove the medicinal twig or medicinal vine. Especially for the patients with hemiplegia，diabetes or weak constitution，and the elderly who are not sensitive to the temperature. During the process of treatment，the doctor should pay attention to the local skin color，it is advisable to make the skin slightly flushed. Excessive，prolonged or intense pressing is avoided during treatment to prevent the scald.

（5）施灸过程中需谨慎，避免引起火灾。

（5）Fire should be prevented cautiously during the process of therapy.

（6）操作后必须交代患者，若施术部位有瘙痒，属正常的治疗反应，避免用手抓破，以免引起感染。6小时内不宜洗澡。

（6）After the operation，the patient should be instructed that itching on the treatment areas is a normal treatment reaction and do not scratch this part. It is not advisable to take a bath within 6 hours.

八、意外情况及处理
Ⅷ　Accidents and handling methods

（1）晕灸。如患者在点灸过程中出现气短、面色苍白、出冷汗等晕灸现象，立即停止操作，让患者头低位平卧，亦可加服少量糖水；若出现严重至昏迷不醒者，立即行急救处理。

（1）Fainting. If the patient develops signs of shortness of breath，pale complexion and cold sweat during ironing，this operation should be stopped immediately，and help the patient lie flat with head-down tilt and drink a small amount of sugar water. If the patient is unconscious，an emergency treatment should be performed immediately.

（2）烫伤、起水疱。如有烫伤，用生理盐水清洁创面并浸润无菌纱布湿敷创面直至疼痛明显减轻或消失后，外涂烧伤膏。如起小水疱，皮肤可自行吸收，保持局部干燥及水疱皮肤的完整性即可；如水疱较大，可用无菌针头将水疱戳破，放出疱内渗液，每天用碘伏消毒，外涂烧伤膏，保持局部干燥及清洁，预防感染。

（2）Scalds and blisters. For Scalds，the surface of the wound should be cleaned with physiological saline and compressed by wet sterile gauzes until the pain is greatly relieved or disappears，and then applied burn ointment. For small blisters，the skin will absorb the blisters fluid if the skin over the blisters is not open and kept dry. For large blisters，a sterile needle can be used to puncture them to release the fluid. The patient should disinfect it with iodophor，apply burn ointment to it，and keep the skin dry and clean every day to prevent infection.

【附注】
【Notes】

药枝或药藤制备
Preparation of Medicinal Twigs or Medicinal Vines

追骨风、牛耳枫、过山香、黑老虎、五味藤、八角枫、当归藤、四方藤、吹风藤适量，均切成 15～20 cm 长的段，晒干，和生姜、大葱、两面针、黄柏、防己一同放入 50 度白酒中浸泡（酒要浸过药面），7 天后取出阴干备用。

The medicinal twigs or medicinal vines include Zhuigufeng（Flos Echinopsis Latifolii），Niuerfeng（Herba Daphniphylli），Guoshanxiang（Radix Litseae Cubebae），Heilaohu（Radix et Caulis Kadsurae Coccineae），Wuweiteng（Caulis Schisandrae Sphenantherae），Bajiaofeng（Radix Alangii），Dangguiteng（*Embelia parviflora* Wall.），Sifangteng（Caulis Cissi），Chuifengteng（Caulis Clematidis et Akebiae）. These medicinal twigs or medicinal vines are cut into long segments in the length of 15 to 20 cm，dried and then soaked in the liquor（50% vol）（liquor should cover these twigs or vines）with ginger，welsh onion，Liangmianzhen （Radix zanthoxyli）, Huangbo（Cortex Phellodendri Chinensis）and Fangji（Radix Stephaniae Tetrandrae）. 7 days later，these twigs or vines will be taken out for shade drying and using.

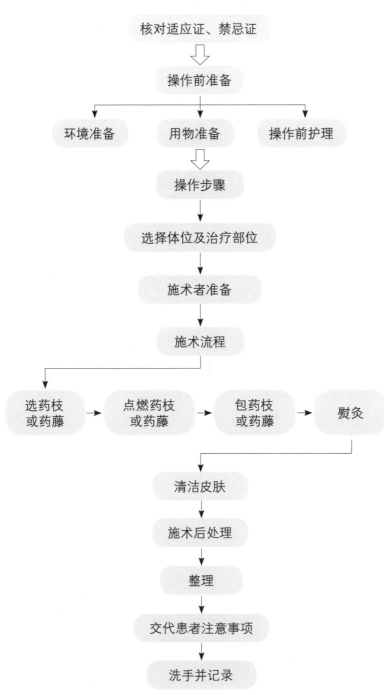

壮医火攻疗法流程图

The Flow Chart about Zhuang Medicine Fire Therapy

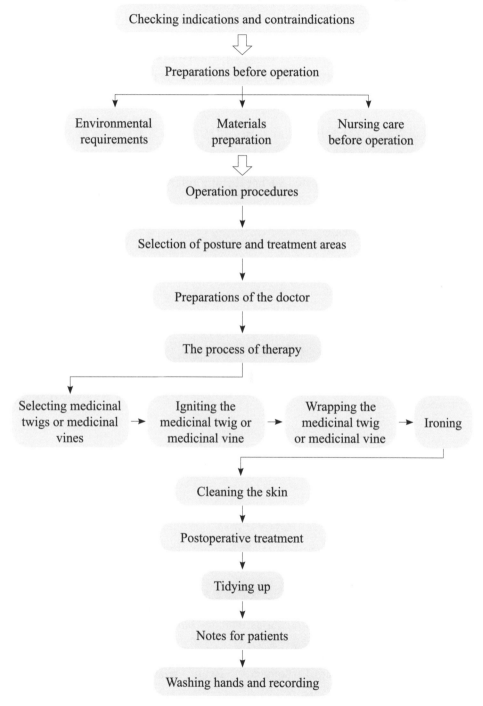

第十章　壮医香囊佩药疗法
Chapter 10　Zhuang Medicine Medicated Sachet Therapy

壮医香囊佩药疗法是用特定壮药加工成药粉放入香囊内，佩系于衣带或身上，通过气道吸收药物有效成分，以治疗疾病的一种方法。

Zhuang medicine medicated sachet therapy refers to a therapeutic method of wearing a sachet filled with the powder of Zhuang medicinal materials and smelling its fragrance to treat diseases.

一、主要功效
Ⅰ　Main effects

通气道，通调龙路、火路，避秽，祛风、湿、瘴等毒。

To regulate airway，dragon route and fire route. To dispel dirty，wind，dampness，miasma，etc.

二、适应证
Ⅱ　Indications

内科、儿科等常见病可使用本疗法治疗，常见适应证有得凉（感冒、上呼吸道感染）、勒爷屙细（小儿泄泻）、勒爷唉疳（小儿疳积）、年闹诺（失眠）、奔浮（水肿）等。

This therapy can be used to treat the common diseases of internal medicine，pediatrics，etc. Its common indications include Deliang（cold，upper respiratory tract infection），Leye'exi（infantile diarrhea），Leyebengan（infantile malnutrition），Niannaonuo（insomnia），Benfu（edema），etc.

三、禁忌证
Ⅲ Contraindications

（1）妊娠期妇女禁用。

（1）It is prohibited for pregnant women.

（2）皮肤过敏者慎用。

（2）It is prohibited for patients suffering from skin sensibility.

四、操作前准备
Ⅳ Preparations before operation

（1）环境要求。治疗室内清洁，安静，光线明亮，温度适宜，避免患者吹风受凉。

（1）Environmental requirements. The treatment room should be clean，quiet and well-lit. Besides，keep the treatment room at an ideal temperature to prevent the patient from catching a cold.

（2）用物准备。药袋（香囊）、药物、压板等（图10-1）。

（2）Materials preparation. Medicine bags（sachets），medicinal materials，a spatula，etc.（Fig. 10-1）.

①药物准备。将选好的药物研磨为细末，密封备用。

① Medicinal materials preparation. The selected medicinal materials should be ground into powder and sealed for later use.

②香囊制作。常用款式为荷包式，选择透气良好的布料制作（图10-2）。

② Sachet-making. The commonly used style is a pouch style design which is made of cloth with good breathability（Fig. 10-2）.

（3）操作前护理。核对患者信息及治疗方案等，说明治疗的意义和注意事项，使患者能积极主动配合操作。

（3）Nursing care before operation. The nurse should check the patient's information and treatment plan，explain the significance and notices of the treatment， enable the patient to cooperate with the doctor for a better operation.

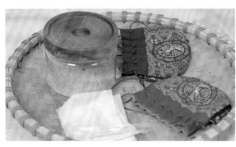

图 10-1 用物准备

Fig. 10-1 Materials preparation

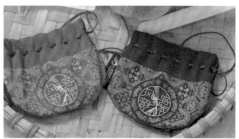

图 10-2 香囊

Fig. 10-2 Sachets

五、操作步骤

V Operation procedures

（1）洗手。

（1）Washing hands.

（2）施术流程。

（2）Operation procedures.

①装药。先将研成末的药物装入小布袋内（图 10-3），一般每个小布袋装药粉 6 g。然后再将小布袋装入香囊中（图 10-4）。

① Putting the herbs powder into the cloth bag. The herb powder is put into a small cloth bag（Fig. 10-3）. In general，each bag contains herbs powder of 6 g. Then，the small cloth bag is put into the sachet（Fig. 10-4）.

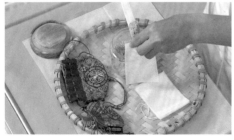

图 10-3 将药物装入小布袋

Fig. 10-3 Putting the herbs powder into a small cloth bag

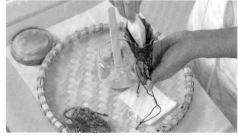

图 10-4 将小布袋装入香囊

Fig. 10-4 Putting the cloth bag into the sachet

②佩挂。根据治疗不同疾病的需要，将香囊佩挂于患者相应的部位。如用于强身，则佩挂于颈部或戴于手腕（图 10-5）；用于防治流行性感冒，则佩挂于颈部、胸前等（图 10-6）；用于保健预防，可佩挂于颈部或置于上衣口袋内，也可挂于室内等，夜间可置于床头（图 10-7）或挂于蚊帐内。

② Wearing the sachet. According to the requirements of treating different diseases, it should be worn on the corresponding parts of the body. If it is used for strengthening physical health, it should be worn around the neck or on the wrist（Fig. 10-5）. If it is used for the prevention and treatment of influenza, it should be worn around the neck or before the chest（Fig. 10-6）. If it is used for health care, it can be worn around the neck and put in the pocket of the jacket. Besides, it can also be hung indoors, placed on the bedside at night（Fig. 10-7）or hung in a mosquito net.

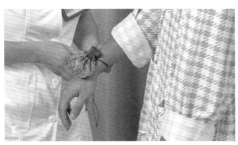

图 10-5　将香囊戴于手腕
Fig. 10-5　Wearing the sachet on the wrist

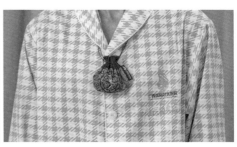

图 10-6　将香囊佩挂于胸前
Fig. 10-6　Wearing the sachet before the chest

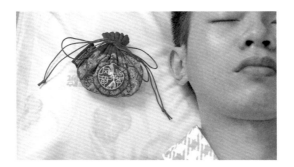

图 10-7　将香囊置于床头
Fig. 10-7　Placing the sachet on the bedside

（3）整理患者衣物及操作物品。

（3）The doctor tidies up the patient's clothing and used materials.

（4）交代患者治疗后注意事项等。

（4）The doctor informs the patient of precautions after treatment.

（5）洗手并记录治疗情况。

（5）The doctor washes hands and makes a record about treatment.

六、疗程
VI　Course of treatment

香囊内药物一般 5 ～ 7 天更换 1 次。壮医香囊佩药疗法一般没有疗程限制，可佩挂至疾病明显好转或痊愈。用于保健预防的药可长期佩挂；若用于避瘟防病，一般以度过传染病流行期为宜。

In general，the herbs powder in the sachet should be changed once every 5 to 7 days. This therapy has no limit to the course of treatment and the sachet can be worn all the time until the disease is significantly improved or cured. The herbs bag for health care and disease prevention can be worn for a long time. The herbs bag for preventing plague can be worn until the end of epidemics.

七、注意事项
VII　Notes

（1）某些外用药有一定的毒性或刺激性，用量过多可引起恶心、呕吐或慢性累积性中毒等。给小儿施用壮医香囊佩药疗法时，注意教育患儿不要随便将袋内药物内服。

（1）Due to the toxicity or irritation of some external medicines，the excessive use of these herbs can cause nausea，vomiting or chronic cumulative poisoning. The doctor should tell children not to take the herbs powder in the sachets orally.

（2）注意保持香囊的干燥，剧烈运动或洗澡时要从身上取下。

（2）Pay attention to keeping the sachet dry and removing it from the body before exercising or taking a bath.

（3）应根据不同的病证需要选择适宜的药物。

（3）The proper medicinal materials should be selected according to different treatment needs.

（4）壮医香囊佩药疗法的主要作用是防病、调病。对于病情较重者，不宜使用本疗法，以免延误治疗时机。

（4）The main function of Zhuang medicine medicated sachet therapy is to prevent and regulate common diseases. This therapy is not suitable for patients with severe diseases so as not to delay the treatment.

八、意外情况及处理
Ⅷ　Accidents and handling methods

患者在佩药过程中如果出现局部皮肤发红、瘙痒、皮疹等过敏现象，应立即停止佩药治疗，严重者立即就医。

If there is redness，itching or rash on the skin during treatment，this therapy should be stopped immediately. If the patient suffers from a severe allergy，he/she needs medical treatment immediately.

【附注】
【Notes】

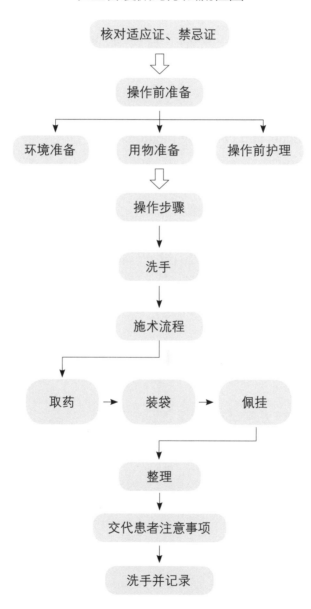

The Flow Chart about Zhuang Medicine Medicated Sachet Therapy

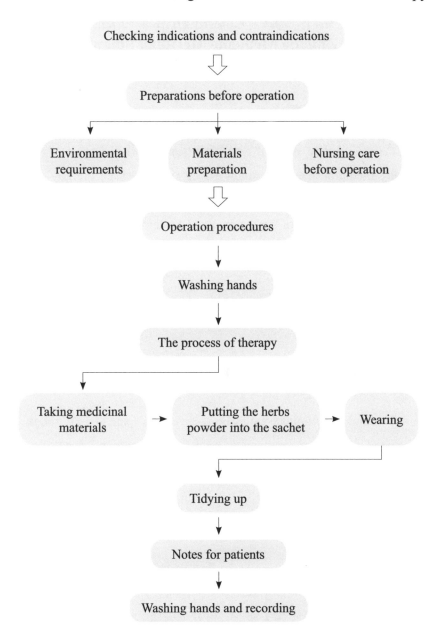

第十一章　壮医经筋推拿疗法
Chapter 11　Zhuang Medicine Meridian Sinew（Jing Jin）Massage Therapy

壮医经筋推拿疗法是在古典十二经筋理论指导下，结合壮族民间理筋术，总结出的将推拿、针刺、拔罐相结合以治疗疾病的一种方法。

Zhuang medicine meridian sinew（Jing jin）massage therapy refers to a therapeutic method of combining manipulation，acupuncture with cupping to treat diseases under the guidance of the theory about tendons along twelve meridians and Zhuang medical soothing tendon manipulation.

一、主要功效
Ⅰ　Main effects

舒筋，解结，消肿，止痛，通痹，祛风、湿、痧、寒、热、瘀等毒，通调三道两路，调节气血平衡。

To relax tendon，eliminate stagnation，swelling，pain and arthralgia spasm. To dispel wind，dampness，pathogen，cold，fever and blood stasis. To regulate three passages and two pathways and the balance between qi and blood.

二、适应证
Ⅱ　Indications

内科、外科、五官科等常见病、多发病均可使用本疗法治疗，常见适应证有发旺（痹病）、甭巧尹（偏头痛）、巧尹（头痛）、活邀尹（颈椎病）、旁巴尹（肩周炎）、核嘎尹（腰腿痛）、麻抹（麻木）、甭裆呷（半身不遂）、年闹诺（失眠）、兰奔（头晕）、林得叮相（跌打损伤）、得凉（感冒、上呼吸道感染）、发得（发热）、奔唉（咳嗽）、胴尹鹿西（腹痛吐泻、急性胃肠炎）、嚎尹（牙痛）、肥胖症等。

This therapy can be used to treat the common diseases and frequently-occurring diseases of internal medicine，surgery，ENT，etc. Its common indications include Fawang（arthralgia disease）, Bengqiaoyin（migraine）, Qiaoyin（headache）, Huoyaoyin（cervical spondylosis）, Pangbayin（scapulohumeral periarthritis）, Hegayin（lumbocrural pain）, Mamo（numbness）, Bengdangxia（hemiplegia）, Niannaonuo（insomnia）, Lanben（dizziness）, Lindedingxiang（traumatic injury）, Deliang（cold, upper respiratory tract infection）, Fade（fever）, Ben'ai（cough）, Dongyinluxi（abdominal pain, vomiting, diarrhea, acute gastroenteritis）, Haoyin（toothache）, obesity, etc.

三、禁忌证
Ⅲ Contraindications

（1）自发出血性疾病患者、凝血功能障碍者禁用。

（1）It is prohibited for patients who suffer from spontaneous hemorrhagic diseases and coagulation disorders.

（2）严重心脑血管疾病患者、血糖控制不佳者、精神病患者、身体极度消瘦虚弱者等禁用。

（2）It is prohibited for patients who have severe cardiovascular and cerebrovascular diseases，poor glycemic control，psychosis，or an extremely weak constitution.

（3）各种骨伤病患者及急性软组织损伤者慎用。

（3）It should be used cautiously for patients who suffer from bone injuries and acute soft tissue injuries.

（4）局部皮肤有破溃、疤痕、高度水肿处及浅表大血管处禁用。

（4）It is prohibited for patients who have skin ulcers，scars or severe edema as well as superficial large vessels.

（5）过度疲劳、过度饥饿、过度饱、醉酒、精神高度紧张的患者禁用。

（5）It is prohibited for patients who suffer from excessive fatigue，excessive hunger，overeating，drunkness or high mental stress.

（6）孕妇禁用。

（6）It is prohibited for pregnant women.

四、操作前准备

Ⅳ　Preparations before operation

（1）环境要求。治疗室内清洁，安静，光线明亮，温度适宜，避免患者吹风受凉。

（1）Environmental requirements. The treatment room should be clean，quiet and well-lit. Besides，keep the treatment room at an ideal temperature to prevent the patient from catching a cold.

（2）用物准备。按摩床、一次性针灸针、复合碘皮肤消毒液、医用棉签或棉球、一次性无菌手套、消毒火罐或真空抽气罐、真空抽气枪、持物钳、治疗巾、打火机、酒精灯等。

（2）Materials preparation. A massage table，disposable acupuncture needles，compound iodine skin disinfectant，medical cotton swabs or cotton balls，disposable sterile gloves，disinfected cupping jars or vacuum air suction cups，a vacuum air suction gun，forceps，treatment towels，a lighter，an alcohol lamp，etc.

（3）操作前护理。核对患者信息及治疗方案等，说明治疗的意义和注意事项，取得患者同意；对患者进行精神安慰与鼓励，消除患者的紧张、恐惧情绪，使患者能积极主动配合操作。

（3）Nursing care before operation. The nurse should check the patient's information and treatment plan and explain the significance and notices of the treatment to obtain the patient's consent. Besides，the nurse should encourage the patient to overcome his/her nervousness and fear and enable the patient to cooperate with the doctor for a better operation.

五、操作步骤

V　Operation procedures

（1）体位选择。根据患者病情确定体位，常取坐位、俯卧位、仰卧位、侧卧位等，以患者舒适及便于施术者操作为宜，避免用强迫体位。

（1）Posture selection. Based on the state of the illness，the posture is selected. Sitting position，prone position，dorsal position or lateral recumbent position is often selected to provide convenience for the patient and the doctor. The compulsive position should be avoided.

（2）部位选择。以痛处为腧，采取"顺藤摸瓜""顺筋摸结"的方法，确定病变所在经筋，查找相关筋结病灶点作为治疗部位。

（2）Position selection. Taking the pain part as the starting point，the doctor can find clues to identify the meridian and tendon where the lesion is located and find the relevant lesion as treatment areas.

（3）洗手。

（3）Washing hands.

（4）施术流程。

（4）Operation procedures.

①手触摸结。采用手触诊察法。两手密切配合，左手着重协助固定诊察部位及提供诊察之便，右手根据所检查部位的生理形态、筋膜的厚薄及层次、正常组织的张力、结构形状等情况，运用拇指的指尖、指腹及拇指与其他四指的指腹握合力（即指合力）（图11-1）或用肘尖（图11-2）作为主要探查工具。指力、撑力、肘力及腰力协调配合，对行检区域（所病经筋循行路线）做浅、中、深层次检查，由浅至深，由轻至重，以循、触、摸（图11-3），按（图11-4），切，拿弹拨（图11-5），推按（图11-6），拨刮（图11-7），钳掐（图11-8），揉捏（图11-9）等手法行检。通过正触觉与异触觉的对比方法，结合患者对检查的反应，识别阳性病灶是否存在及其表现的特征、所处的部位、与周围组织的关系等。

① Finding the lesion by palpation. Palpation is used. Treatment areas are fixed by the left hand for providing convenience for the examination. According to the physiological form of the part to be examined，the thickness and layer of the tendons，the tension，structure and shape of the normal tissue，the way of combining the tip and pulp of the thumb with the resultant force of five fingers of the right hand（Fig. 11-1）or the olecranon（Fig. 11-2）is used for examination. Finger force，support force，elbow force and lumbar force are used to examine the related part（the running course of meridian for this disease）with palpation（Fig. 11-3），pressing（Fig. 11-4），poking channels manipulation（Fig. 11-5），pushing manipulation（Fig. 11-6），scraping manipulation（Fig. 11-7），pinching manipulation（Fig. 11-8）or malaxation（Fig. 11-9）from mild strength to intense strength.Through the comparison of normal and abnormal tactile sensation as well as the patient's response to the examination，the doctor can identify positive lesions and their characteristics，location and the relationship with surrounding tissues.

②手法解结。先用肘滚法（图 11-10）在病变部位来回滚动 3 ～ 5 遍，使局部充分放松发热。再将肘部和手指相结合，顺着病变部位的经筋线实施按（图 11-4）、揉捏（图 11-9）、点（图 11-11）、推按（图 11-6）、捏拿（图 11-12）等分经理筋手法，施术时间 15 ～ 20 分钟。

② Manipulations to treat the tendon node. The rolling manipulation with the elbow（Fig. 11-10）is used on the lesion 3 to 5 times to fully relax it. Soothing tendon manipulations including pressing（Fig. 11-4），malaxation（Fig. 11-9），point pressing manipulation（Fig. 11-11），pushing（Fig. 11-6），and kneading manipulation（Fig. 11-12）are performed along the running course of meridian of lesion part with the elbow and fingers. The operation lasts 15 to 20 minutes.

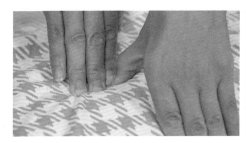

图 11-1　指合力摸结
Fig. 11-1　Touching the tendon node with the resultant force of fingers

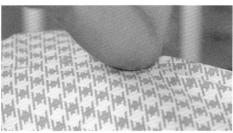

图 11-2　肘尖探结
Fig. 11-2　Touching the tendon node with the olecranon

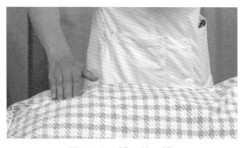

图 11-3　循、触、摸

Fig. 11-3　Palpation

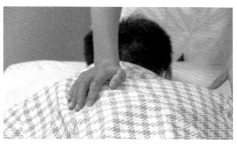

图 11-4　按

Fig. 11-4　Pressing manipulation

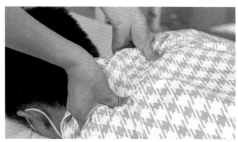

图 11-5　拿弹拨

Fig. 11-5　Poking channels manipulation

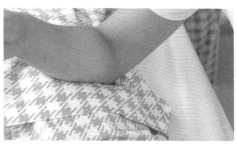

图 11-6　推按

Fig. 11-6　Pushing manipulation

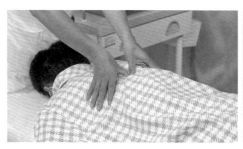

图 11-7　拨刮

Fig. 11-7　Scraping manipulation

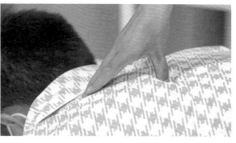

图 11-8　钳掐

Fig. 11-8　Pinching manipulation

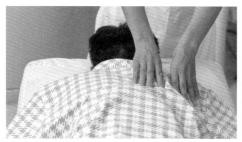

图 11-9　揉捏

Fig. 11-9　Malaxation

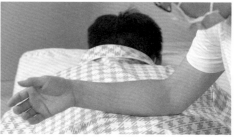

图 11-10　肘滚法

Fig. 11-10　Rolling manipulation with the elbow

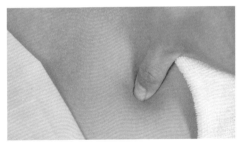 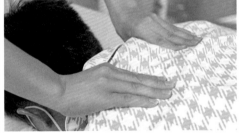

图 11-11 点   图 11-12 捏拿

Fig. 11-11 Point pressing manipulation   Fig. 11-12 Kneading manipulation

③针刺除结。

③ Acupuncture to treat the tendon node.

洗手，戴一次性无菌手套。

The doctor washes hands and wears disposable sterile gloves.

消毒。用具消毒。选择一次性针灸针、消毒火罐或真空抽气罐（图 11-13）进行消毒。部位消毒。常规消毒施术部位皮肤，消毒范围的直径大于施术部位 5 cm。

Disinfection. Disinfection of materials. Disposable acupuncture needles，disinfected cupping jars or vacuum air suction cups（Fig. 11-13）are chosen for disinfection. Skin disinfection. The skin of treatment areas is disinfected and the diameter of the disinfection area is larger than that of treatment areas（exceeding 5 cm）.

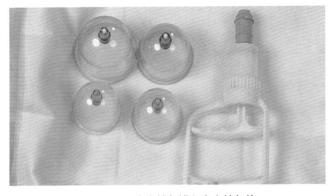

图 11-13 真空抽气罐和真空抽气枪

Fig. 11-13 Vacuum air suction cups and a vacuum air suction gun

固结行针。施术者一手持一次性针灸针（一般选用规格为0.4 mm×40 mm），另一手拇指按压固定查及的筋结点，根据筋结的大小、部位深浅进行探刺，使气达病所后快速出针，可一孔多针、一针多向，不留针。

Pressing the tendon node and using a needle. The doctor holds a disposable acupuncture needle（usually 0.40 mm×40 mm）with one hand，and presses and fixes the tendon node with the thumb of the other hand. Besides，the doctor needs to perform the acupuncture according to the size and location of tendon node，and then withdraws the needle quickly after qi reaching the affected part. The method of multi-needle on one tendon node or multi-direction with one needle can be used and no needle is left.

注意：如为寒证，可用壮医火针疗法。局部常规消毒，施术者左手拇指按压固定查及的筋结点，右手持火针针具，将针尖置于酒精灯上烧红至发白（图11-14），迅速将针尖垂直刺入皮肤，直达筋结点，不留针。

Note：Zhuang medicine fire-needle therapy can be used for the cold syndrome. The doctor disinfects the local skin，presses and fixes the tendon node with the left thumb，holds the fire needle with the right hand，and then puts the needle tip on an alcohol lamp to burn until it turns white（Fig. 11-14）. Finally，the doctor inserts the needle vertically into the tendon node at a fast speed and no needle is left.

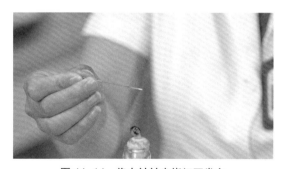

图 11-14　将火针针尖烧红至发白
Fig. 11-14　Burning the needle tip until it turns white

④施罐散结。

④ Cupping to eliminate the tendon node.

拔罐。在针刺筋结点上拔罐（图11-15），留罐5～10分钟，以拔出黄水为佳。

Cupping. Cupping is performed on the tendon node（Fig. 11-15）and lasts for 5 to 10 minutes. It is better to pull out the yellow water.

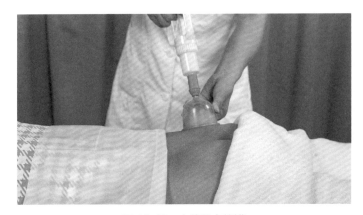

图 11-15　在筋结点拔罐
Fig. 11-15　Cupping on the tendon node

起罐。将真空抽气罐活塞拔起，然后把罐向一侧倾斜，让空气进入罐内，慢慢将罐提起，用医用棉签或棉球擦拭所拔部位流出的黄水或血液，常规消毒治疗部位的皮肤。

Removal of the cups. The doctor pulls up the piston of the vacuum air suction cup，tilts the cup to one side，lets the air flow into the cup，and then slowly lifts the cup and cleans the yellow water or blood at treatment areas with a medical cotton swab or cotton ball. Besides，the skin at this area is routinely disinfected.

（5）施术后处理。冲洗火罐或真空抽气罐内瘀血并放入含氯消毒液中浸泡，后送消毒供应中心统一消毒。

（5）Postoperative treatment. The doctor cleans the blood stasis in the cupping jars or vacuum air suction cups，places them in chlorine-containing disinfectant，and then sends them to the central sterile supply department to prevent cross infection.

（6）整理患者衣物及操作物品。

（6）The doctor tidies up the patient's clothing and used materials.

（7）交代患者治疗后注意事项等。

（7）The doctor informs the patient of precautions after treatment.

（8）洗手并记录治疗情况。

（8）The doctor washes hands and makes a record about treatment.

六、疗程
Ⅵ　Course of treatment

每天 1 次，10 次为 1 个疗程。

Once a day，10 times as a course of treatment.

七、注意事项
Ⅶ　Notes

（1）患者过度疲劳、过度饥饿、过度饱、精神高度紧张时不能操作。暴露治疗部位时，应注意保护患者隐私及保暖。

（1）It is prohibited for patients who suffer from excessive fatigue，excessive hunger，overeating or high mental stress. When treatment areas are exposed，the doctor should protect the patient's privacy and keep the patient warm.

（2）严格执行无菌技术操作，防止感染。

（2）Aseptic operation should be implemented strictly to prevent infection.

（3）施术者选择好合适的位置、步态、姿势，以利于发力和持久操作，并避免自身劳损。

（3）The doctor adopts the appropriate position，gait，and posture for long-lasting operation to avoid self-injury.

（4）施术时注意患者状况，操作细致，手法由轻到重，宜使用巧力，不可粗暴用力，以防造成患者损伤。注意留罐时间，避免出现水疱。

（4）Pay attention to the patient's condition during the operation. The doctor should perform the operation meticulously and use the force flexibly from mild manipulation to intense manipulation to prevent damage. Pay attention to the time of cupping to avoid blisters.

（5）手触摸结时，对一时难以辨认的病灶，需多次复检或做会诊检查及特殊检查。对可疑细菌性感染、恶性变等异态病灶，需及时做相应检查，以鉴别确诊。

（5）When the lesion can't be identified temporarily by palpation，the doctor should do several re-examinations，or have a consultation or special examination. The corresponding examinations should be carried out on abnormal lesions such as suspected bacterial infection and malignant transformation to identify and diagnose them.

（6）治疗后避免患者立即起身离开，为其安排舒适体位，嘱其休息 5 ～ 10 分钟后方可活动。

（6）Prevent the patient from getting up and leaving immediately after treatment. Let the patient take a comfortable posture and rest for 5 to 10 minutes.

（7）嘱患者拔罐后切勿使局部受风受凉，4 ～ 6 小时内禁止洗澡。

（7）Tell the patient not to expose treatment areas to wind after cupping and do not take a bath within 4 to 6 hours.

（8）操作后应清淡饮食，忌食辛辣、油炸、刺激食物。

（8）The patient should eat a bland diet after treatment，foods that are spicy，greasy and stimulating should be avoided.

八、意外情况及处理
VIII　Accidents and handling methods

（1）晕针、晕罐。如患者治疗过程中出现气短、面色苍白、出冷汗等晕针现象，立即让患者头低位平卧，亦可加服少量糖水；若出现严重至昏迷不醒者，立即行急救处理。

（1）Fainting. If the patient develops shortness of breath，pale complexion and cold sweat，this operation should be stopped immediately，and help the patient lie flat with head-down tilt and drink a small amount of sugar water. If the patient is unconscious，an emergency treatment should be performed immediately.

（2）血肿。用消毒干棉球按压血肿部位针孔 3 ～ 5 分钟，防止血肿变大；出血量较大的血肿可加以冷敷，以促进凝血，24 小时后可行热敷，促进血肿吸收。

（2）Hematoma. The pinhole of the hematoma part should be pressed with a disinfected dry cotton ball for 3 to 5 minutes to avoid larger hematoma. The hematoma with a large amount of blood should be treated with cold compress firstly to promote coagulation and the hot compress after 24 hours to promote the absorption of hematoma.

（3）烫伤、起水疱。如有烫伤，用生理盐水清洁创面并浸润无菌纱布湿敷创面直至疼痛明显减轻或消失后，外涂烧伤膏。如起小水疱，皮肤可自行吸收，保持局部干燥及水疱皮肤的完整性即可；如水疱较大，可用无菌针头将水疱戳破，放出疱内渗液，每天用碘伏消毒，外涂烧伤膏，保持局部干燥及清洁，预防感染。

（3）Scalds and blisters. For scalds，the surface of the wound should be cleaned with physiological saline and compressed by wet sterile gauzes until the pain is greatly relieved or disappears，then applied with burn ointment. For small blisters，the skin will absorb the blisters fluid if the skin over the blisters is not open and kept dry. For large blisters，a sterile needle can be used to puncture them to release the fluid. The patient should disinfect it with iodophor and apply burn ointment to it. Besides，the patient should keep the skin dry and clean every day to prevent infection.

【附注】
【Notes】

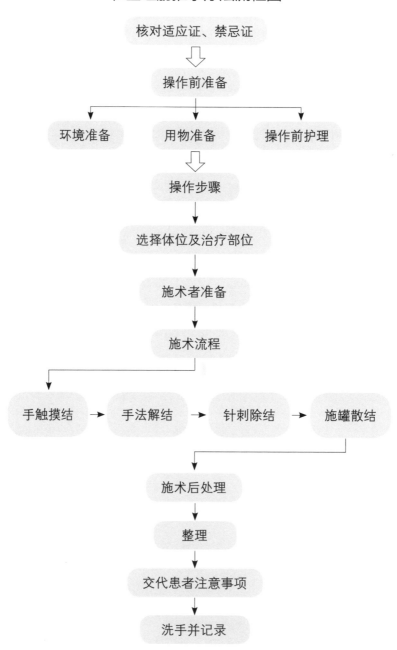

壮医经筋推拿疗法流程图

核对适应证、禁忌证

⬇

操作前准备

环境准备　　用物准备　　操作前护理

⬇

操作步骤

选择体位及治疗部位

施术者准备

施术流程

手触摸结 → 手法解结 → 针刺除结 → 施罐散结

施术后处理

整理

交代患者注意事项

洗手并记录

The Flow Chart about Zhuang Medicine Meridian Sinew（Jing Jin）Massage Therapy

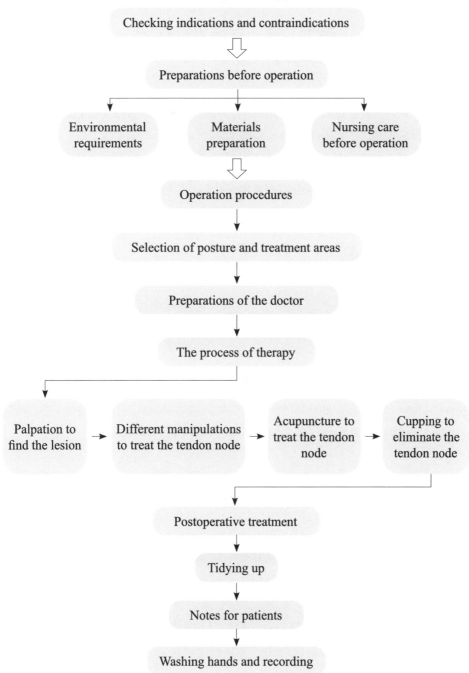

第十二章 壮医火针疗法
Chapter 12 Zhuang Medicine Fire-Needle Therapy

壮医火针疗法是在壮医理论指导下，将针具的针尖烧红至发白后，迅速刺入穴位或特定部位，以治疗疾病的一种方法。

Zhuang medicine fire-needle therapy refers to a therapeutic method of puncturing acupoints or specific parts quickly after burning the needle tip until it turns white under the guidance of Zhuang medicine theory.

一、主要功效
I Main effects

祛风、湿、痧、寒、痰、瘀等毒，消肿，散结，通痹，止痛，通调三道两路，调节气血平衡。

To dispel wind, dampness, pathogen, cold, phlegm and blood stasis. To eliminate swelling, stagnation, arthralgia spasm and pain. To regulate three passages and two pathways, and the balance between qi and blood.

二、适应证
II Indications

内科、外科、妇科、儿科、五官科、皮肤科等常见病、多发病均可使用本疗法治疗，常见适应证有贫痧（痧症）、发旺（痹病）、核嘎尹（腰腿痛）、活邀尹（颈椎病）、旁巴尹（肩周炎）、骆芡（骨性关节炎）、隆芡（痛风）、麻抹（麻木）、甭裆呷（半身不遂）、林得叮相（跌打损伤）、年闹诺（失眠）、巧尹（头痛）、奔呗啷（带状疱疹、带状疱疹后遗神经痛）、能啥累（瘙痒、湿疹）、叻仇（痤疮）等。

This therapy can be used to treat the common diseases and frequently-occurring diseases of internal medicine, surgery, gynecology, pediatrics, ENT, dermatology, etc. Its common indications include Pinsha (acute filthy disease), Fawang (arthralgia disease), Hegayin (lumbocrural pain), Huoyaoyin (cervical spondylosis), Pangbayin (scapulohumeral periarthritis), Luoqian (osteoarthritis), Longqian (gout), Mamo (numbness), Bengdangxia (hemiplegia), Lindedingxiang (traumatic injury), Niannaonuo (insomnia), Qiaoyin (headache), Benbeilang (shingles, postherpetic neuralgia), Nenghanlei (pruritus, eczema), Lechou (acne), etc.

三、禁忌证
Ⅲ　Contraindications

（1）自发出血性疾病患者、凝血功能障碍者禁用。

（1）It is prohibited for patients who suffer from spontaneous hemorrhagic diseases and coagulation disorders.

（2）严重心脑血管疾病患者、血糖控制不佳者、精神病患者、身体极度消瘦虚弱者等禁用。

（2）It is prohibited for patients who have severe cardiovascular and cerebrovascular diseases, poor glycemic control, psychosis, or an extremely weak constitution.

（3）局部皮肤有破溃、疤痕、高度水肿处及浅表大血管处禁用。

（3）It is prohibited for patients who have skin ulcers, scars or severe edema as well as superficial large vessels.

（4）过度疲劳、过度饥饿、过度饱或精神高度紧张的患者禁用。

（4）It is prohibited for patients who suffer from excessive fatigue, excessive hunger, overeating or high mental stress.

（5）孕妇禁用。

（5）It is prohibited for pregnant women.

四、操作前准备

IV   Preparations before operation

（1）环境要求。治疗室内清洁，安静，光线明亮，温度适宜，避免患者吹风受凉。

（1）Environmental requirements. The treatment room should be clean, quiet and well-lit. Besides, keep the treatment room at an ideal temperature to prevent the patient from catching a cold.

（2）用物准备。一次性针灸针（一般选用规格为 0.4 mm×40 mm，可根据患者病情及病位选择不同规格的针具）、一次性无菌手套、复合碘皮肤消毒液、医用棉签或棉球、打火机、酒精灯。

（2）Materials preparation. Disposable acupuncture needles（usually 0.4 mm×40 mm, different sizes of needles can be selected according to the patient's disease condition and treatment areas）, disposable sterile gloves, compound iodine skin disinfectant, medical cotton swabs or cotton balls, a lighter, an alcohol lamp.

（3）操作前护理。核对患者信息及治疗方案等，说明治疗的意义和注意事项，取得患者同意；对患者进行精神安慰与鼓励，消除患者的紧张、恐惧情绪，使患者能积极主动配合操作。

（3）Nursing care before operation. The nurse should check the patient's information and treatment plan and explain the significance and notices of the treatment to obtain the patient's consent. Besides, the nurse should encourage the patient to overcome his/her nervousness and fear and enable the patient to cooperate with the doctor for a better operation.

五、操作步骤

V   Operation procedures

（1）体位选择。根据患者病情确定体位，常取坐位、俯卧位、仰卧位、侧卧位等，以患者舒适及便于施术者操作为宜，避免用强迫体位。

（1）Posture selection. Based on the state of illness, the posture is selected. Sitting position, prone position, dorsal position or lateral recumbent position is often selected to provide convenience for the patient and the doctor. The compulsive position should be avoided.

（2）部位选择。根据病证选取适当的治疗穴位或特定部位。

（2）Position selection. According to the disease patterns, the corresponding acupoint or specific part is selected.

（3）施术流程。

（3）Operation procedures.

①经筋摸结。运用拇指的指尖、指腹及拇指与其他四指的指合力，或用肘尖，对经筋循行路线做浅、中、深层次检查，由浅至深，由轻至重，以切、循、按、摸、弹拨、推按、拨刮、钳掐、揉捏等手法行检。筋结分点、线、面等形状，触摸有粗糙样、小颗粒状、结节状、条索状、线样甚至成片状，大小不一，深浅不一，以触压疼痛异常敏感为特征。

① Finding tendon nodes along the running course of meridian. The way of combining the tip and pulp of the thumb with the resultant force of five fingers or the olecranon is used to examine the related part（the running course of meridian of this disease）with massage, pressing manipulation, palpation, poking channels manipulation, pushing manipulation, scraping manipulation, pinching manipulation or kneading manipulation from mild strength to intense strength. The shapes of tendon nodes include point, line, plane, etc. The doctor can feel that tendon nodes are rough, granular, nodular, cord-like, line-like or even flaky in different sizes and depths. It is characterized by pain and abnormal sensitivity after pressing.

②火针消结。

② Fire the needles to eliminate tendon nodes.

洗手，戴医用外科口罩、医用帽子和一次性无菌手套。

The doctor washes hands, and wears a surgical mask, a medical cap and disposable sterile gloves.

消毒。针具消毒。选择一次性针灸针（图 12-1）并进行常规消毒。部位消毒。常规消毒施术部位皮肤，消毒范围的直径大于施术部位 5 cm。

Disinfection. Needle disinfection. Disposable acupuncture needles（Fig. 12-1）are chosen for routine disinfection. Skin disinfection. The skin of treatment areas is disinfected and the diameter of disinfection area is larger than that of treatment areas （exceeding 5 cm）.

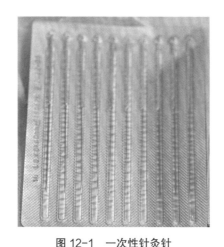

图 12-1　一次性针灸针

Fig. 12-1　Disposable acupuncture needles

施针。施术者以左手按压固定查及的筋结点（图 12-2），右手持火针针具，将针尖置于酒精灯上烧红直至发白（图 12-3），根据筋结的大小、部位深浅迅速将针尖垂直刺入皮肤，直达筋点，疾进疾出（图 12-4、图 12-5），不留针，每个筋结点施针 3 ～ 5 次。

Performing acupuncture. The doctor presses and fixes the tendon node（Fig. 12-2）with the left hand，holds the fire needle with the right hand，and then puts the needle tip on an alcohol lamp to burn until it turns white（Fig. 12-3）. Finally，the doctor inserts the needle vertically into the tendon node at a fast speed （Fig. 12-4，Fig. 12-5）according to its size and location. No needle is left and acupuncture 3 to 5 times should be performed on each tendon node.

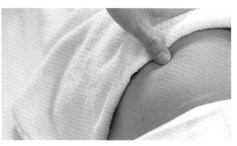

图 12-2　摸节查灶

Fig. 12-2　Pressing the tendon node to find the lesion

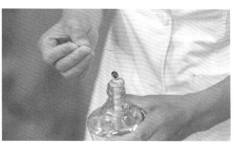

图 12-3　烧红针尖直至发白

Fig. 12-3　Burning the needle tip until it turns white

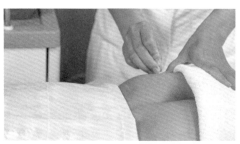

图 12-4　疾进

Fig. 12-4　Inserting the needle quickly

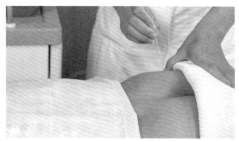

图 12-5　疾出

Fig. 12-5　Withdrawing the needle quickly

（4）施术后处理，用过的针具置于利器盒中销毁处理。

（4）The used needles should be put in a sharps box after operation.

（5）整理患者衣物及操作用品。

（5）The doctor tidies up the patient's clothing and used materials.

（6）交代患者治疗后注意事项等。

（6）The doctor informs the patient of precautions after treatment.

（7）洗手并记录治疗情况。

（7）The doctor washes hands and makes a record about treatment.

六、疗程

VI　Course of treatment

隔天 1 次，7 ～ 10 次为 1 个疗程。

Once every other day，7 to 10 times as a course of treatment.

七、注意事项

VII　Notes

（1）患者过度疲劳、过度饥饿、过度饱或精神高度紧张时不能操作。暴露治疗部位时，应注意保护患者隐私及保暖。治疗过程中随时观察患者局部皮肤及病情，随时询问患者的耐受程度，防止患者晕针。

（1）It is prohibited for patients who suffer from excessive fatigue, excessive hunger, overeating or high mental stress. When treatment areas are exposed, the doctor should protect the patient's privacy and keep the patient warm. During this process, the doctor should observe the skin and patient's condition as well as ask the patient's tolerance to this therapy at any time.

（2）根据患者体质和病情，注意掌握刺激手法和刺激强度。

（2）Pay attention to mastering the manipulation and stimulating intensity according to the patient's constitution and disease condition.

（3）操作过程中应小心、谨慎、迅速，进针深浅适度，避免损伤龙路、火路及内脏。

（3）Be careful, cautious, and agile during the operation. The inserting depth should be moderated to avoid the damage to the dragon route, fire route and internal organs.

（4）治疗过程中应遵守无菌操作规则，防止感染。

（4）Aseptic operation should be obeyed during treatment to prevent infection.

（5）交代患者若施术部位有瘙痒，属正常的治疗反应，避免用手抓破，以免引起感染。6小时内不宜洗澡。

（5）After the operation, the patient should be instructed it is normal if there is itching in treatment areas, do not scratch this part. It is not advisable to take a bath within 6 hours.

（6）治疗后在饮食上应注意忌口（如各种皮肤病患者，在针刺治疗期间忌食发物），以清淡饮食为主。

（6）Diet should be paid attention to after the treatment. The patient who has skin diseases should avoid eating stimulating food and eat a bland diet during treatment.

八、意外情况及处理

VIII　Accidents and handling methods

（1）晕针。如患者治疗过程中出现气短、面色苍白、出冷汗等晕针现象，立即让患者头低位平卧，亦可加服少量糖水；若出现严重至昏迷不醒者，立即行急救处理。

（1）Fainting. If the patient develops shortness of breath，pale complexion and cold sweat，this operation should be stopped immediately，and help the patient lie flat with head-down tilt and drink a small amount of sugar water. If the patient is unconscious，an emergency treatment should be performed immediately.

（2）血肿。用消毒干棉球按压血肿部位针孔 3 ～ 5 分钟，防止血肿变大；出血量较大的血肿可加以冷敷，以促进凝血。

（2）Hematoma. The pinhole of the hematoma part should be pressed with a disinfected dry cotton ball for 3 to 5 minutes to avoid larger hematoma. The hematoma with a large amount of blood should be treated with cold compress first to promote coagulation.

【附注】
【Notes】

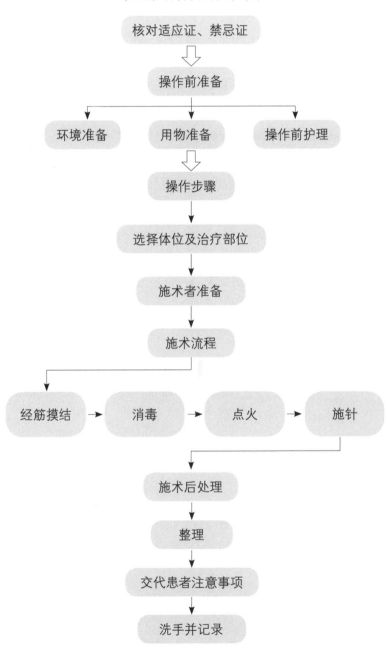

壮医火针疗法流程图

The Flow Chart about Zhuang Medicine Fire-Needle Therapy

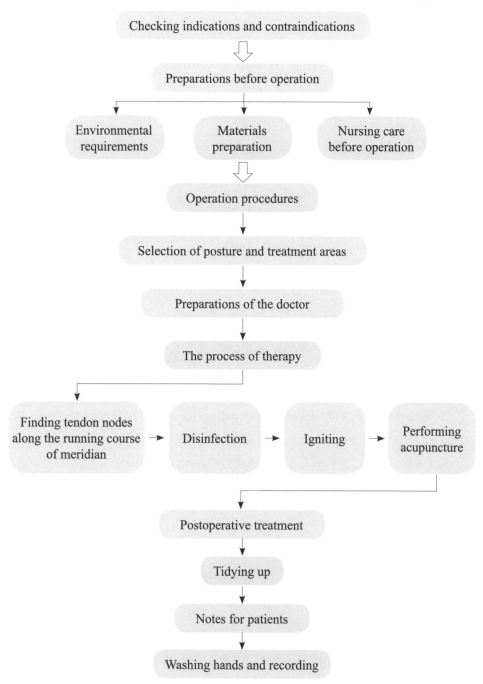

第十三章　壮医针挑疗法
Chapter 13　Zhuang Medicine Needle-Pricking Therapy

壮医针挑疗法是使用针具通过不同挑刺手法，挑破浅表皮肤反应点，挑出皮下纤维，以通龙路、火路，调三道气机，逐瘀毒外出，进而治疗疾病的一种方法。

Zhuang medicine needle-pricking therapy refers to a therapeutic method of using needles to prick the skin reactive points and pick out the subcutaneous fibers through different pricking methods to regulate three passages and two pathways, the balance between qi and blood and dispel stasis.

一、主要功效
Ⅰ　Main effects

祛风、寒、热、湿、痧、瘴、痰等毒，消肿，散结，通痹，通调三道两路，调节气血平衡。

To dispel wind, cold, fever, dampness, pathogen, miasma and phlegm. To eliminate swelling, stagnation, and arthralgia spasm. To regulate three passages and two pathways, and the balance between qi and blood.

二、适应证
Ⅱ　Indications

内科、外科、妇科、儿科、五官科、皮肤科等常见病、多发病均可使用本疗法治疗，常见适应证有贫痧（痧症）、啰尹（疼痛）、发旺（痹病）、活邀尹（颈椎病）、核尹（腰痛）、巧尹（头痛）、林得叮相（跌打损伤）、麻邦（中风）、麻抹（麻木）、奔墨（哮喘）、奔唉（咳嗽）、胴尹（胃痛）、京尹（痛经）、啰呗啷（带状疱疹、带状疱疹后遗神经痛）、能啥累（瘙痒、湿疹）、呗仇（痤疮）等。

This therapy can be used to treat the common diseases and frequently-occurring diseases of internal medicine, surgery, gynecology, pediatrics, ENT, dermatology, etc. Its common indications include Pinsha (acute filthy disease), Benyin (pain), Fawang (arthralgia disease), Huoyaoyin (cervical spondylosis), Heyin (low back pain), Qiaoyin (headache), Lindedingxiang (traumatic injury), Mabang (stroke), Mamo (numbness), Benmo (asthma), Ben'ai (cough), Dongyin (stomachache), Jingyin (dysmenorrhea), Benbeilang (shingles, postherpetic neuralgia), Nenghanlei (pruritus, eczema), Lechou (acne), etc.

三、禁忌证
Ⅲ　Contraindications

（1）自发出血性疾病患者、凝血功能障碍者禁用。

（1）It is prohibited for patients who suffer from spontaneous hemorrhagic disease and coagulation disorders.

（2）严重心脑血管疾病患者、血糖控制不佳者、精神病患者、身体极度消瘦虚弱者等禁用。

（2）It is prohibited for patients who have severe cardiovascular and cerebrovascular diseases, poor glycemic control, psychosis, or an extremely weak constitution.

（3）精神病患者，精神高度紧张、狂躁不安、抽搐不能合作者禁用。

（3）It is prohibited for patients who suffer from psychosis, high mental stress, mania, anxiety, or spasm.

（4）局部皮肤有破溃、疤痕、高度水肿处及浅表大血管处禁用。

（4）It is prohibited for patients who have skin ulcers, scars or severe edema as well as superficial large vessels.

（5）过度疲劳、过度饥饿、过度饱或极度虚弱者禁用。

（5）It is prohibited for patients who suffer from excessive fatigue, excessive hunger，overeating or an extremely weak constitution.

（6）孕妇禁用。

（6）It is prohibited for pregnant women.

四、操作前准备
Ⅳ Preparations before operation

（1）环境要求。治疗室内清洁，安静，光线明亮，温度适宜，避免患者吹风受凉。

（1）Environmental requirements. The treatment room should be clean，quiet and well-lit. Besides，keep the treatment room at an ideal temperature to prevent the patient from catching a cold.

（2）用物准备。一次性无菌注射器针头或三棱针、手术刀片、复合碘皮肤消毒液、医用棉签、无菌纱布、消毒真空抽气罐或玻璃罐、大浴巾、一次性无菌手套等。

（2）Materials preparation. Disposable sterile syringe needles or three-edged needles，a knife blade，compound iodine skin disinfectant，medical cotton swabs，sterile gauzes，disinfected vacuum air suction cups or glasses，large bath towels，disposable sterile gloves，etc.

（3）操作前护理。核对患者信息及治疗方案等，说明治疗的意义和注意事项，取得患者同意；对患者进行精神安慰与鼓励，消除患者的紧张、恐惧情绪，使患者能积极主动配合操作。

（3）Nursing care before operation. The nurse should check the patient's information and treatment plan and explain the significance and notices of the treatment to obtain the patient's consent. Besides，the nurse should encourage the patient to overcome his/her nervousness and fear and enable the patient to cooperate with the doctor for a better operation.

五、操作步骤

V　Operation procedures

（1）体位选择。根据患者病情确定体位，常取俯卧位、仰卧位、侧卧位等，以患者舒适及便于施术者操作为宜，避免用强迫体位。

（1）Posture selection. Based on the state of the illness，the posture is selected. Prone position，dorsal position or lateral recumbent position is often selected to make patients feel comfortable and doctors feel easy to operate. The compulsive position should be avoided.

（2）部位选择。根据病证选取相应的治疗部位，避开浅表大血管。

（2）Position selection. According to the disease patterns，the corresponding acupoint or specific part is selected and the superficial large blood vessels should be avoided.

（3）洗手，戴医用外科口罩、医用帽子和一次性无菌手套。

（3）The doctor should wash hands，then，wear a surgical mask，a medical cap and disposable sterile gloves.

（4）消毒。

（4）Disinfection.

①针具消毒。选择一次性注射器针头（7号针头：0.7 mm×32 mm）或三棱针（图 13-1）并进行常规消毒。

① Needle disinfection. Disposable syringe needles（size 7 needle：0.7 mm×32 mm）or disinfected three-edged needles（Fig. 13-1）are chosen for routine disinfection.

②部位消毒。用复合碘皮肤消毒液常规消毒施术部位皮肤，消毒范围的直径大于施术部位 5 cm（图 13-2）。

② Skin disinfection. The related skin is disinfected with compound iodine skin disinfectant and the diameter of the disinfection area is larger than that of treatment areas（exceeding 5 cm）（Fig. 13-2）.

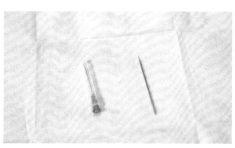

图 13-1　一次性注射器针头（左）和三棱针（右）

Fig. 13-1　A disposable syringe needle（left）
and a three-edged needle（right）

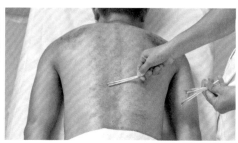

图 13-2　部位消毒

Fig. 13-2　Skin disinfection

（5）施术流程。

（5）Operation procedures.

①选挑点。一般选取皮肤反应点或阿是穴作为挑点。

① Selection of pricking point. In general，the skin reactive point or Ashi acupoint is selected as pricking point.

②持针。左手食指轻压挑点一侧以固定皮肤，右手拇指、食指、中指三指持针身，露出针尖 1 ～ 2 cm（图 13-3），无名指在针尾上部支持和调节运针（图 13-4）。

② Needle holding. One side of the pricking point is pressed lightly by the left index finger to fix skin，the needle body is held by the right thumb，index finger and middle finger，and the needle tip is exposed by 1 to 2 cm（Fig. 13-3）. Then，the upper part of the needle end is supported and adjusted by the ring finger（Fig. 13-4）.

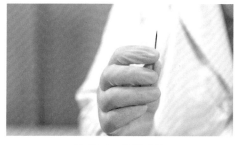

图 13-3　持针手势

Fig. 13-3　Gesture of needle holding

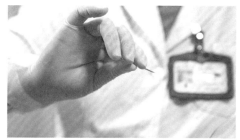

图 13-4　持针手势

Fig. 13-4　Gesture of needle holding

③行针。初下针时，持针要稳定，用力要均匀，不可用力太猛。针身与皮肤成 30° 角（图 13-5），对准挑点迅速入针，针尖挑着皮下纤维适当地用沉劲以无名指压低针身，提高针尖向上挑起，挑出或挑断皮下组织中白色纤维状物质。

③ Needle inserting. When the needle is inserted into the pricking point，the needle should be held stably，and the force should be steady and moderate. Firstly，the needle is held at a 30° angle to the skin（Fig. 13-5）and inserted into the pricking point quickly. Secondly， subcutaneous fibers are pricked by the needle tip. Finally，the body of the needle is pressed down properly by the ring finger to let the needle tip be raised for picking out white fibrous material in subcutaneous tissue.

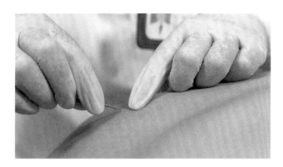

图 13-5　与皮肤表面成 30° 角进针
Fig. 13-5　Needle inserting at a 30° angle to the skin

④摆针。在挑治过程中，如纤维较粗，可先将皮下白色纤维状物质拉至针口，然后一边做前后摇摆，一边向上用力缓慢拉出纤维（图 13-6）。反复挑尽挑点周围（以挑点为中心，直径 0.5 ～ 1 cm 范围）的皮下纤维，顺序由上往下。如挑出的纤维较多而不易挑断时，可用手术刀片割断（图 13-7），随挑随割。

④ Needle swinging. If the fibers are thick in the process of pricking，the doctor can pull the white fibrous material in subcutaneous tissue to the pinhole，then，swing them back and forth and pull out the fibers slowly（Fig. 13-6）. All the subcutaneous fibers around the point are pricked（taking the pricking point as the center with a diameter of 0.5 to 1 cm as the pricking area）from top to bottom. If there are too many fibers which are not easy to break，the doctor can cut them with a knife blade（Fig. 13-7）.

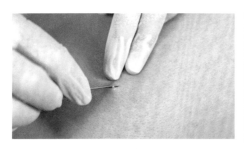

图 13-6 摆针

Fig. 13-6   Needle swinging

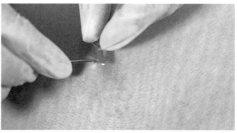

图 13-7 割断纤维

Fig. 13-7   Cutting fibers

⑤施罐。

⑤ Cupping operation.

拔罐。挑尽所有挑点的纤维，依据患者病情可在挑点处予以拔罐，留罐 10 ~ 15 分钟（图 13-8），并盖上大浴巾。

Cupping. All the subcutaneous fibers around the pricking point are pricked. According to the patient's disease condition，cupping can be performed at the pricking point and last for 10 to 15 minutes（Fig. 13-8）and a large bath towel should be used to cover it.

起罐。将真空抽气罐活塞拔起，慢慢将罐提起（图 13-9），用无菌纱布擦拭所拔部位。

Removal of the cup. The doctor pulls up the piston of the vacuum air suction cup and slowly lifts the cup and cleans the treatment area with sterile gauzes（Fig. 13-9）.

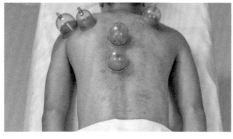

图 13-8 拔罐

Fig. 13-8   Cupping

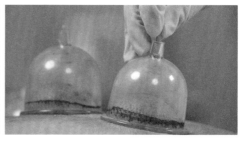

图 13-9 起罐

Fig. 13-9   Removal of the cup

⑥术毕，常规消毒所有针挑点。

⑥ After the operation，all pricking points are routinely disinfected.

（6）施术后处理。将注射器针头或三棱针丢入利器盒。冲洗真空抽气罐内瘀血后放入消毒液中浸泡消毒。

（6）Postoperative treatment. The used syringe needles or three-edged needles should be thrown into the sharps box. The doctor cleans the blood stasis in the vacuum air suction cups and places them in the disinfectant.

（7）整理患者衣物及操作物品。

（7）The doctor tidies up the patient's clothing and used materials.

（8）交代患者治疗后注意事项等。

（8）The doctor informs the patient of precautions after treatment.

（9）洗手并记录治疗情况。

（9）The doctor washes hands and makes a record about treatment.

六、疗程
Ⅵ　Course of treatment

一般每次挑 8～10 个点，3～5 天 1 次，5～7 次为 1 个疗程。

In general，8 to 10 points are pricked each time，once every 3 to 5 days，5 to 7 times as a course of treatment.

七、注意事项
Ⅶ　Notes

（1）患者过度疲劳、过度饥饿、过度饱、精神高度紧张或极度虚弱时不能操作。暴露治疗部位时，应注意保护患者隐私及保暖。

（1）It is prohibited for patients who suffer from excessive fatigue，excessive hunger，overeating，high mental stress or an extremely weak constitution. When treatment areas are exposed，the doctor should protect the patient's privacy and keep the patient warm.

（2）患者最好取卧位，以防晕针。

（2）The patient should take the supine position to prevent fainting during pricking.

（3）持针的手指不能拿在针体过前或过后的部位，以免下针时用力不均匀，影响疗效和污染针尖。

（3）When inserting the needle，the doctor should hold the middle part of the needle to avoid uneven force which affects the curative effect and contaminates the needle tip.

（4）施术宜轻、巧、准、疾，刺入深浅要适度，避免损伤患者内脏，针头切忌在皮下乱刺、乱戳。施术过程中避开浅表大血管，随时观察患者局部皮肤及病情，随时询问患者对针挑的耐受程度。

（4）The operation should be mild，skillful，accurate，and fast. The depth of needle inserting should be moderate to avoid the damage to patient's internal organs. During this process，the doctor should avoid superficial large vessels and observe the skin and patient's condition as well as ask the patient's tolerance to this therapy at any time.

（5）操作后必须交代患者，局部皮肤会出现红晕或红肿，挑治后有热痛感，停止针挑 1 ～ 2 周左右可自行消失。若出现局部发痒，避免用手搔抓针挑口，以免引起感染；若不小心抓破，不必惊慌，注意保持清洁，用复合碘皮肤消毒液消毒即可。针挑后当日不宜做重活，注意休息。

（5）The doctor must instruct the patient that the local skin will appear flushed or swollen and there will be heat pain after pricking，which will disappear on its own in 1 to 2 weeks after stopping the therapy. If there is itching on the local skin，the patient should avoid scratching the pinhole to avoid infection；don't panic，keep it clean，and disinfect it with compound iodine skin disinfectant after scratching. It is not advisable for patients to do heavy work on the same day and patients should pay attention to resting.

（6）消毒必须严格，保持施术部位皮肤清洁干燥，24 小时内不宜洗澡，以防伤口感染。

（6）The doctor should strictly perform disinfection and keep the skin of treatment areas clean and dry. It is not advisable for patients to take a bath within 24 hours to avoid wound infection.

（7）治疗期间患者应清淡饮食，避免进食辛辣等刺激性食物。

（7）The patient should eat a bland diet during treatment and avoid spicy foods.

八、意外情况及处理

Ⅷ　Accidents and handling methods

（1）晕针。如患者在治疗过程中出现气短、面色苍白、出冷汗等晕针现象，立即停止操作，让患者头低位平卧，亦可加服少量糖水；若出现严重至昏迷不醒者，立即行急救处理。

（1）Fainting. If the patient develops shortness of breath，pale complexion and cold sweat，this operation should be stopped immediately，and help the patient lie flat with head-down tilt and drink a small amount of sugar water. If the patient is unconscious，an emergency treatment should be performed immediately.

（2）针挑后，局部呈红晕或红肿未能完全消失时，保持针孔清洁，可用复合碘皮肤消毒液消毒，预防感染；极少数患者会出现针孔部位红肿情况，告知患者注意保持局部清洁，不要擦伤针孔，局部涂红霉素软膏以防感染加重，必要时到医院进一步处理。

（2）The local skin will appear flushed or swollen after pricking，the patient should keep the pinhole clean and disinfect it with compound iodine skin disinfectant to prevent infection. Few patients may suffer from skin redness and swelling around the pinhole，the doctor should instruct the patient that they should keep treated areas clean and apply erythromycin ointment to prevent the infection from worsening，and go to the hospital for further treatment if necessary.

【附注】
【Notes】

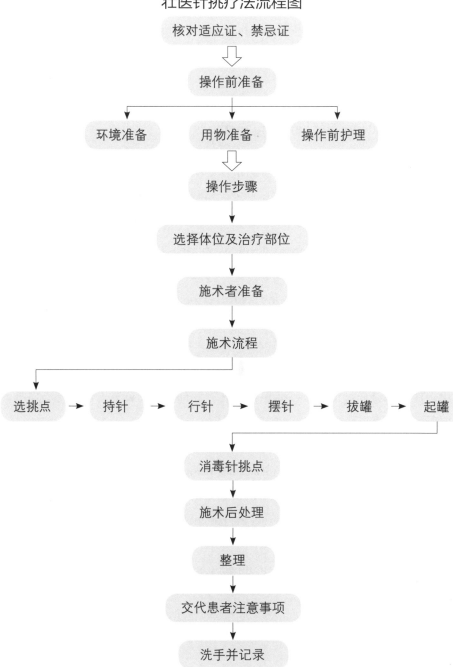

壮医针挑疗法流程图

核对适应证、禁忌证
⬇
操作前准备

环境准备　　用物准备　　操作前护理
⬇
操作步骤
⬇
选择体位及治疗部位
⬇
施术者准备
⬇
施术流程

选挑点 → 持针 → 行针 → 摆针 → 拔罐 → 起罐
⬇
消毒针挑点
⬇
施术后处理
⬇
整理
⬇
交代患者注意事项
⬇
洗手并记录

The Flow Chart about Zhuang Medicine Needle-Pricking Therapy

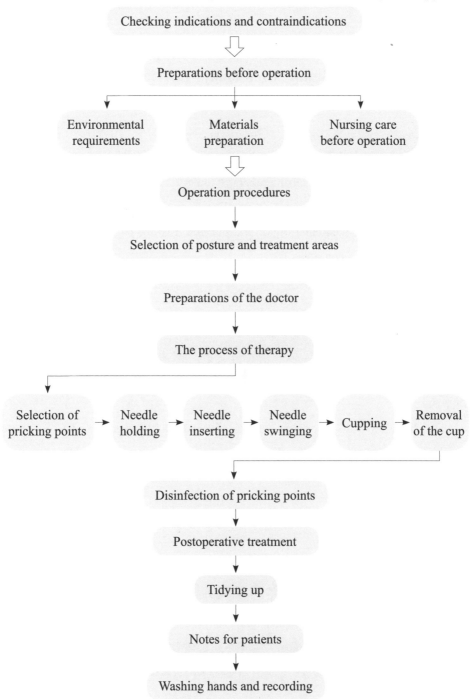

第十四章　壮医包药疗法
Chapter 14　Zhuang Medicinal Materials Bag Therapy

壮医包药疗法是将壮药饮片或鲜品研成粉或捣碎后，用特制药酒调和，装入纱袋，取冷药或热药包敷于患处，以治疗疾病的一种方法。

Zhuang medicinal materials bag therapy refers to a therapeutic method of using Zhuang medicine decoction pieces or grinding fresh medicinal materials which are blended with special medicinal liquor and put into a gauze bag to treat the affected part with a cold or hot compress.

一、主要功效
Ⅰ　Main effects

祛风、湿、寒、热、瘀等毒，消肿，散结，止痛，通调三道两路，调节气血平衡。

To dispel wind, dampness, cold, fever and blood stasis. To eliminate swelling, stagnation, and pain. To regulate three passages and two pathways, and the balance between qi and blood.

二、适应证
Ⅱ　Indications

内科、外科、妇科、儿科、五官科、皮肤科等常见病、多发病等均可使用本疗法治疗，常见适应证有夺扼（骨折）、林得叮相（跌打损伤）、发旺（痹病）、隆芡（痛风）、呗哝（痈疮肿痛）、额哈（虫蛇咬伤）、麻抹（麻木）、嗪佛（包块肿块）、旁巴尹（肩周炎）、活邀尹（颈椎病）、夺核拖（腰椎间盘突出症）、产后腊胴尹（产后腹痛）、京尹（痛经）、兵嘿细勒（疝气）、北嘻（乳腺炎）、航靠谋（腮腺炎）等。

This therapy can be used to treat the common diseases and frequently-occurring diseases of internal medicine, surgery, gynecology, pediatrics, ENT, dermatology, etc. Its common indications include Duo'e（fracture）, Lindedingxiang（traumatic injury）, Fawang（arthralgia disease）, Longqian（gout）, Beinong（ulcerative carbuncle, swelling and pain）, Eha（insect or snake bites）, Mamo（numbness）, Benfo（lump）, Pangbayin（scapulohumeral periarthritis）, Huoyaoyin（cervical spondylosis）, Duohetuo（lumbar disc herniation）, postpartum Ladongyin（postpartum abdominal pain）, Jingyin（dysmenorrhea）, Bingheixile（hernia）, Beixi（mastitis）, Hangkaomou（parotitis）, etc.

三、禁忌证
Ⅲ　Contraindications

（1）局部皮肤破溃、高度水肿、开放性骨折、外伤出血者禁用。

（1）It is prohibited for patients who have skin ulcers, severe edema, open fracture and bleeding wound.

（2）孕妇慎用。

（2）It is prohibited for pregnant women.

四、操作前准备
Ⅳ　Preparations before operation

（1）环境要求。治疗室内清洁，安静，光线明亮，温度适宜，避免患者吹风受凉。

（1）Environmental requirements. The treatment room should be clean, quiet and well-lit. Besides, keep the treatment room at an ideal temperature to prevent the patient from catching a cold.

（2）用物准备。

（2）Materials preparation.

①药袋、药粉（图14-1）、药酒或小青柠檬（图14-2）。

① Medicinal materials bags，medicinal powder（Fig. 14-1），medicinal liquor or small green lemons（Fig. 14-2）.

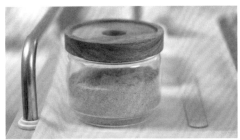
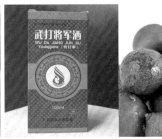

图 14-1　药粉

Fig. 14-1　Medicinal powder

图 14-2　药酒（左）和小青柠檬（右）

Fig. 14-2　Medicinal liquor（left）and small green lemons（right）

②绷带或胶布、防水小铺巾、剪刀、复合碘皮肤消毒液、纱布袋、生理盐水、消毒棉签和棉球、一次性无菌莲花针、一次性无菌手套、消毒真空抽气罐、真空抽气枪。

② Bandages or adhesive plaster，waterproof drapes，scissors，compound iodine skin disinfectant，gauze bags，physiological saline，sterile cotton swabs and cotton balls，disposable sterile lotus needles，disposable sterile gloves，disinfected vacuum air suction cups and a vacuum air suction gun.

（3）操作前护理。核对患者信息及治疗方案等，说明治疗的意义和注意事项，取得患者同意；对患者进行精神安慰与鼓励，消除患者的紧张、恐惧情绪，使患者能积极主动配合操作。

（3）Nursing care before operation. The nurse should check the patient's information and treatment plan and explain the significance and notices of the treatment to obtain the patient's consent. Besides，the nurse should encourage the patient to overcome his/her nervousness and fear and enable the patient to cooperate with the doctor for a better operation.

五、操作步骤
V　Operation procedures

（1）体位选择。根据患者病情确定体位，常取坐位、俯卧位、仰卧位、侧卧位等，以患者舒适及便于施术者操作为宜，避免用强迫体位。

（1）Posture selection. Based on the state of the illness，the posture is selected. Sitting position，prone position，dorsal position or lateral recumbent position is often selected to provide convenience for the patient and the doctor. The compulsive position should be avoided.

（2）洗手，戴医用外科口罩、医用帽子和一次性无菌手套。

（2）The doctor should wash hands，and wear a surgical mask，a medical cap and disposable sterile gloves.

（3）清洁。用消毒棉球蘸生理盐水清洁治疗部位的皮肤（图14-3）。

（3）Cleaning. Clean the skin of treatment areas with sterile cotton balls and physiological saline（Fig. 14-3）.

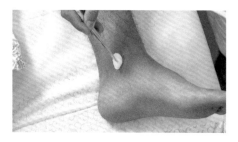

图 14-3　清洁皮肤
Fig. 14-3　Cleaning the skin

（4）施术流程。

（4）Operation procedures.

①按包药部位大小取适量药粉，加特制药酒或小青柠檬汁（图14-4）调和适中，置于纱布袋内，封口备用。阳证取冷敷（图14-5）；阴证取热敷，需将药物炒热或用微波炉加热（图14-6）。

① According to the size of the treatment areas，the doctor takes an appropriate amount of medicinal powder，blends it with special medicinal liquor or small green lemon juice（Fig. 14-4）, and then puts it in a gauze bag to seal it for later use. Cold compress is used for Yang syndrome（Fig. 14-5）. Hot compress is used for Yin syndrome and medicinal powder needs to be heated（Fig. 14-6）.

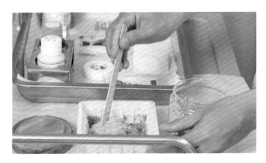

图 14-4　调药

Fig. 14-4　Blending medicinal powder with special medicinal liquor or small green lemon juice

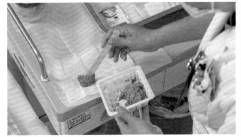 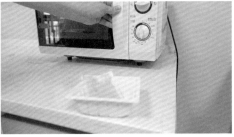

图 14-5　阳证冷敷　　　　　　　　　　图 14-6　加热药物

Fig. 14-5　Cold compress for Yang syndrome　　　Fig. 14-6　Heating medicinal powder

②待药包温度适宜（不超过 45 ℃）后包敷于患处（图 14-7），用绷带或胶布加以固定（图 14-8）。

② When the temperature of the medicinal materials bag is suitable（<45 ℃）, the doctor applies it to the affected part（Fig. 14-7）and fixes it with a bandage or adhesive plaster（Fig. 14-8）.

③患处存在瘀血、肿胀、疼痛明显者，可行壮医莲花针拔罐逐瘀疗法后（图 14-9）再予包敷。

③ For patients with obvious swelling and pain due to blood stasis, the doctor should apply Zhuang medicine stasis-removing therapy with lotus-needling and cupping（Fig. 14-9）before this therapy.

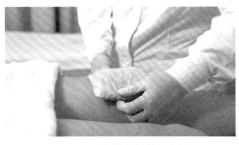

图 14-7 将药包包敷于患处
Fig. 14-7 Applying the medicinal materials bag to the affected part

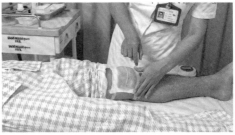

图 14-8 固定药包
Fig. 14-8 Fixing the medicinal materials bag

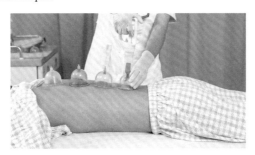

图 14-9 壮医莲花针拔罐逐瘀疗法
Fig. 14-9 Zhuang medicine stasis-removing therapy with lotus-needling and cupping

（5）整理患者衣物及操作物品。

（5）The doctor tidies up the patient's clothing and used materials.

（6）交代患者治疗后注意事项等。

（6）The doctor informs the patient of precautions after treatment.

（7）洗手并记录治疗情况。

（7）The doctor washes hands and makes a record about treatment.

六、疗程
Ⅵ Course of treatment

每天 1 次，10 天为 1 个疗程，一般持续 1 ～ 3 个疗程，每个疗程间隔时间不宜超过 3 天。

Once a day，10 days as a course of treatment，1 to 3 courses of treatment. The time interval between courses of treatment should not exceed 3 days.

七、注意事项

VII　Notes

（1）暴露治疗部位时，应注意保护患者隐私及保暖。治疗过程中随时观察患者局部皮肤及病情，随时询问患者耐受程度。

（1）When treatment areas are exposed, the doctor should protect the patient's privacy and keep the patient warm. During this process, the doctor should observe the patient's skin and condition as well as ask the patient's tolerance to this therapy at any time.

（2）注意患者对药包温度的耐受程度，若温度过高，则可待其降到适宜温度时再进行治疗。

（2）Pay attention to the patient's tolerance to the temperature of the medicinal materials bag. If the temperature is too high, the doctor can perform the treatment after it is at a normal temperature.

（3）若为闭合性骨折移位患者，应先行骨折复位术；若为开放性骨折患者，应待伤口愈合无感染后方可施治。

（3）For patients who suffer from closed fracture displacement, reduction of fracture should be performed first. For patients who suffer from open fractures, this therapy can not be used until the wound heals without infection.

（4）注意掌握包药的松紧度，以免造成局部循环障碍或导致内包药物漏出从而降低疗效和污染衣物。

（4）Pay attention to the elasticity of the operation to avoid local disturbance of blood circulation or leakage of the medicinal powder which will reduce the efficacy and contaminate clothing.

（5）嘱患者严格遵循敷贴时间，儿童不宜超过 1 小时，成人 2～4 小时，不宜擅自延长时间。

（5）The doctor should instruct the patient to strictly follow the treatment time which should not exceed 1 hour for children and 2 to 4 hours for adults.

（6）换药时注意观察患部皮肤颜色的变化，一旦发生破溃要采取适当方法处理，以减少对皮肤的损害。

（6）The doctor should pay attention to the changes in the skin color of the affected part when changing dressings. Once ulceration occurs，proper measures should be taken to reduce the damage to the skin.

（7）必须交代患者在包药期间注意治疗部位的感觉，如包药后皮肤出现瘙痒难耐、灼热、疼痛等感觉时，应立即取下药包，并禁止抓挠，注意保持患部清洁，不宜擅自涂抹别的药物，一般轻症可自愈；若皮肤出现红肿、水疱、破溃等严重反应，须及时到医院就诊。

（7）The doctor should instruct the patient to pay attention to the feeling about treatment areas during the treatment. If there is itching，burning，and pain on the skin，the medicinal materials bag should be removed immediately. Besides，do not scratch and pay attention to keeping skin clean. It is not advisable to apply other ointments because mild symptoms can be self-cure. If the skin has severe reactions such as redness，swellings，blisters，or ulcerations，it is necessary to go to the hospital in time.

（8）根据自身病情，患者治疗后在饮食上应注意忌口（如忌食生冷、油腻、发物等），以清淡饮食为主。

（8）According to the disease condition，the patient should avoid eating cold dishes，oily food and stimulating food. The patient should eat a bland diet after treatment.

八、意外情况及处理
Ⅷ　Accidents and handling methods

如有烫伤，用生理盐水清洁创面并浸润无菌纱布湿敷创面直至疼痛明显减轻或消失后，外涂烧伤膏。如起小水疱，皮肤可自行吸收，保持局部干燥及水疱皮肤的完整性即可；如水疱较大，可用无菌针头将水疱戳破，放出疱内渗液，每天用碘伏消毒，外涂烧伤膏，保持局部干燥及清洁，预防感染。

For scalds，the surface of the wound should be disinfected with physiological saline and compressed by wet sterile gauzes until the pain is greatly relieved or disappears，and then applied burn ointment.For small blisters，the skin will absorb the blisters fluid if the skin over the blisters is not open and kept dry. For large blisters，a sterile needle can be used to puncture them to release the fluid. The patient should disinfect it with iodophor and apply burn ointment to it. Besides，the patient should keep the skin dry and clean every day to prevent infection.

【附注】
【Notes】

壮医包药疗法常用组方

Commonly Used Formulas for Zhuang Medicinal Materials Bag Therapy

根据不同病证选用方剂，取干品饮片打粉或鲜品捣碎备用。

Different formulas are selected according to different disease patterns. The doctor can grind Zhuang medicine decoction pieces or fresh medicinal materials for later use.

（1）夺扼（骨折）、林得叮相（跌打损伤）。方药组成：乳香、没药、伸筋草、威灵仙、桂枝、艾叶、凤仙透骨草、鸡血藤、骨碎补、乌药等。

（1）Duo'e（fracture），Lindedingxiang（traumatic injury）. Formula composition：Ruxiang（Olibanum），Moyao（Myrrha），Shenjincao（Herba Lycopodii），Weilingxian（Radix et Rhizoma Clematidis），Guizhi（Ramulus Cinnamomi），Aiye（Folium Artemisiae Argyi），Fengxiantougucao（Caulis Impatientis Balsaminae），Jixueteng（Caulis Spatholobi），Gusuibu（Rhizoma Drynariae），Wuyao（Radix Linderae），etc.

（2）发旺（痹病）、隆芡（痛风）。

（2）Fawang（arthralgia disease），Longqian（gout）.

①阴证方药组成：红木香、黑老虎、战骨、南蛇藤、千年健、车前草、姜黄、莪术、威灵仙、冰片等。

① The formula composition of Yin syndrome：Hongmuxiang（Radix Kadsurae Longipedunculatae），Heilaohu（Radix et Caulis Kadsurae Coccineae），Zhangu

（Caulis Premnae Fulvae）, Nansheteng（Radix et Caulis Celastri Orbiculati）, Qiannianjian（Rhizoma Homalomenae）, Cheqiancao（Herba Plantaginis）, Jianghuang（Rhizoma Curcumae Longae）, Ezhu（Rhizoma Curcumae）, Weilingxian（Radix et Rhizoma Clematidis）, Bingpian（Borneolum Syntheticum）, etc.

②阳证方药组成：薜荔果、络石藤、穿破石、豨莶草、地不容、石膏、姜黄、宽筋藤、车前草、冰片等。

② The formula composition of Yang syndrome：Biliguo（Fructus Fici Pumilae）, Luoshiteng（Caulis et Folium Trachelospermi）, Chuanposhi（Radix Cudraniae Cochinchinensis）, Xixiancao（Herba Siegesbeckiae）, Diburong（Radix Stephaniae Epigaeae）, Shigao（Gypsum Fibrosum）, Jianghuang（Rhizoma Curcumae Longae）, Kuanjinteng（Caulis Tinosporae Sinensis）, Cheqiancao（Herba Plantaginis）, Bingpian（Borneolum Syntheticum）, etc.

（3）呗哝（痈疮肿痛）。

（3）Beinong（ulcerative carbuncle, swelling and pain）.

方药组成：杠板归、水杨梅、叶下珠、五爪金龙、积雪草、赛葵、三白草、半枝莲、冰片等。

Formula composition：Gangbangui（Herba Polygoni Perfoliati）, Shuiyangmei（Herba Adinae Rubellae）, Yexiazhu（Herba Phyllanthi Urinariae）, Wuzhaojinlong（Radix seu Herba Tetrastigmatis Hypoglauci）, Jixuecao（Herba Centellae）, Saikui（Herba Malvastri Coromandeliani）, Sanbaicao（Herba Saururi）, Banzhilian（Herba Scutellariae Barbatae）, Bingpian（Borneolum Syntheticum）, etc.

（4）额哈（虫蛇咬伤）。

（4）Eha（insect or snake bites）.

方药组成：杠板归、七叶一枝花、葎草、叶下珠、虫牙药、田基黄、乌云盖雪、地不容、半枝莲等。

Formula composition：Gangbangui（Herba Polygoni Perfoliati）, Qiyeyizhihua（Rhizoma Paridis Chinensis）, Lvcao（Herba Humuli Scandentis）, Yexiazhu（Herba Phyllanthi Urinariae）, Chongyayao（Herba seu Folium Rabdosiae Ternifoliae）, Tianjihuang（Herba Hyperici Japonici）, Wuyungaixue（Radix Rubi Parvifolii）, Diburong（Radix Stephaniae Epigaeae）, Banzhilian（Herba Scutellariae Barbatae）, etc.

（5）唪佛（包块肿块）。

（5）Benfo（lump）.

方药组成：杠板归、五爪金龙、姜黄、莪术、瓜蒌、芒硝等。

Formula composition：Gangbangui（Herba Polygoni Perfoliati）, Wuzhaojinlong（Radix seu Herba Tetrastigmatis Hypoglauci）, Jianghuang（Rhizoma Curcumae Longae）, Ezhu（Rhizoma Curcumae）, Gualou（Fructus Trichosanthis）, Mangxiao（Natrii Sulfas）, etc.

（6）北嘻（乳腺炎）、航靠谋（腮腺炎）。

（6）Beixi（mastitis）, Hangkaomou（parotitis）.

方药组成：臭牡丹、粪箕笃、鸡骨草、旱田草、重楼、姜黄、莪术、瓜蒌、芒硝等。

Formula composition：Choumudan（Caulis et Folium Clerodendri Bungei）, Fenjidu（Herba Stephaniae Longae）, Jigucao（Herba Abri）, Hantiancao（Herba Linderniae Ruellioidis）, Chonglou（Rhizoma Paridis）, Jianghuang（Rhizoma Curcumae Longae）, Ezhu（Rhizoma Curcumae）, Gualou（Fructus Trichosanthis）, Mangxiao（Natrii Sulfas）, etc.

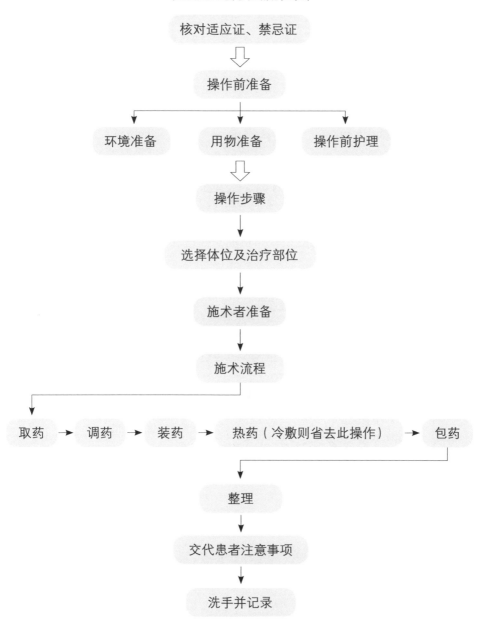

壮医包药疗法流程图

The Flow Chart about Zhuang Medicinal Materials Bag Therapy

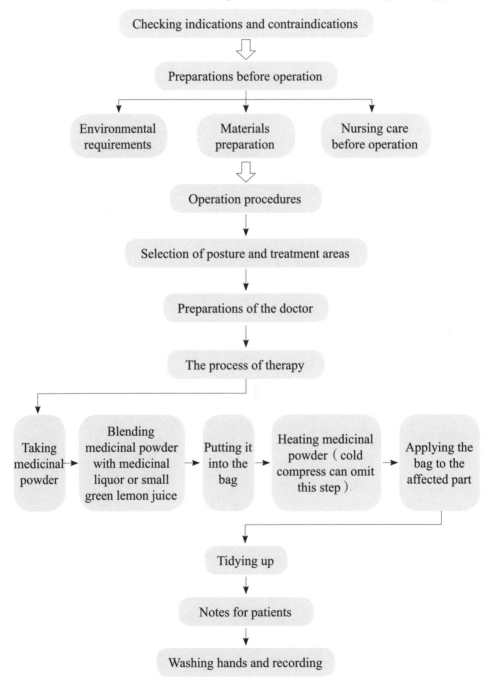

第十五章 壮医全身药浴疗法
Chapter 15 Zhuang Medicine Whole Body Medicated Bath Therapy

壮医全身药浴疗法是用单味或复方壮药，煎汤取液，选择适宜温度，进行全身洗浴，以治疗疾病的一种方法。

Zhuang medicine whole body medicated bath therapy refers to a therapeutic method of decocting single or compound medicinal materials to bathe the whole body at a suitable temperature.

一、主要功效
Ⅰ Main effects

祛风、湿、痧、瘴、热、寒、痰、瘀等毒，消肿，止痒，止痛，活血，温经，补虚，通调三道两路，调节气血平衡。

To dispel wind，dampness，pathogen，miasma，fever，cold，phlegm and blood stasis. To eliminate swelling，itching and pain. To promote blood circulation，warm the meridians and restore deficiency. To regulate three passages and two pathways，and the balance between qi and blood.

二、适应证
Ⅱ Indications

内科、外科、妇科、儿科、五官科、皮肤科等常见病、多发病均可使用本疗法治疗，常见适应证有贫痧（痧症）、能啥累（瘙痒、湿疹）、唪呗啷（带状疱疹、带状疱疹后遗神经痛）、夺扼（骨折）、林得叮相（跌打损伤）、发旺（痹病）、隆芡（痛风）、麻抹（麻木）、唪佛（包块肿块）、旁巴尹（肩周炎）、活邀尹（颈椎病）、核嘎尹（腰腿痛）、产后腊胴尹（产后腹痛）、京尹（痛经）、约京乱（月经不调）、卟很裆（不孕）、盆腔炎、兵嘿细勒（疝气）、北嘻（乳腺炎）等。

This therapy can be used to treat the common diseases and frequently-occurring diseases of internal medicine, surgery, gynecology, pediatrics, ENT, dermatology, etc. Its common indications include Pinsha（acute filthy disease）, Nenghanlei（pruritus, eczema）, Benbeilang（shingles, postherpetic neuralgia）, Duo'e（fracture）, Lindedingxiang（traumatic injury）, Fawang（arthralgia disease）, Longqian（gout）, Mamo（numbness）, Benfo（lump）, Pangbayin（scapulohumeral periarthritis）, Huoyaoyin（cervical spondylosis）, Hegayin（lumbocrural pain）, postpartum Ladongyin（postpartum abdominal pain）, Jingyin（dysmenorrhea）, Yuejingluan（irregular menstruation）, Buhendang（infertility）, pelvic inflammatory disease, Bingheixile（hernia）, Beixi（mastitis）, etc.

三、禁忌证
Ⅲ Contraindications

（1）严重心脑血管疾病患者、血糖控制不佳者、精神病患者、身体极度消瘦虚弱者等禁用。

（1）It is prohibited for patients who have severe cardiovascular and cerebrovascular diseases, poor glycemic control, psychosis, or an extremely weak constitution.

（2）局部皮肤破溃、高度水肿、开放性骨折、外伤出血者禁用。

（2）It is prohibited for patients who have skin ulcers, severe edema, open fracture and bleeding wounds.

（3）过度疲劳、过度饥饿、过度饱或精神高度紧张的患者禁用。

（3）It is prohibited for patients who suffer from excessive fatigue, excessive hunger, overeating or high mental stress.

（4）孕妇慎用。

（4）It is prohibited for pregnant women.

四、操作前准备
Ⅳ　Preparations before operation

（1）环境要求。治疗室内清洁，安静，光线明亮，温度适宜，避免患者吹风受凉。

（1）Environmental requirements. The treatment room should be clean，quiet and well-lit. Besides，keep the treatment room at an ideal temperature to prevent the patient from catching a cold.

（2）用物准备。

（2）Materials preparation.

①药物。根据患者病情选择相应药物，加水煮药，取药液备用（图 15-1）。

① Zhuang medicinal materials. According to the patient's disease condition，corresponding medicinal materials are decocted and the liquid medicine is taken out for later use（Fig. 15-1）.

②其他用物。泡浴大木桶、一次性泡浴袋、浴巾（图 15-2）。

② Other materials. A large wooden barrel for bathing，a disposable bath bag，and bath towels（Fig. 15-2）.

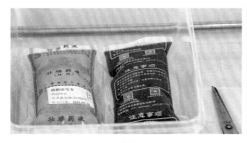
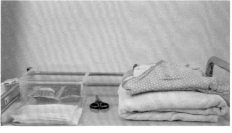

图 15-1　配好的药液
Fig. 15-1　Prepared liquid medicine

图 15-2　其他用物
Fig. 15-2　Other materials

（3）操作前护理。核对患者信息及治疗方案等，说明治疗的意义和注意事项，取得患者同意；对患者进行精神安慰与鼓励，消除患者的紧张、恐惧情绪，使患者能积极主动配合操作。

（3）Nursing care before operation. The nurse should check the patient's information and treatment plan and explain the significance and notices of the treatment to obtain the patient's consent. Besides, the nurse should encourage the patient to overcome his/her nervousness and fear and enable the patient to cooperate with the doctor for a better operation.

五、操作步骤
V   Operation procedures

（1）体位选择。全身药浴常取坐位，避免用强迫体位。

（1）Posture selection. The patient should take a sitting position when taking a whole body medicated bath and a compulsive position should be avoided.

（2）消毒。采用一次性泡浴袋，一人一袋。

（2）Disinfection. One disposable bath bag for one person.

（3）施术流程。

（3）Operation procedures.

①放药。垫好一次性泡浴袋（图 15-3），将药液倒入泡浴大木桶内（图 15-4），药液量以能淹没浴者胸部（取坐姿）为宜。

① Putting the liquid medicine into the large wooden barrel. The disposable bath bag is put in a large wooden barrel（Fig. 15-3），and then liquid medicine is poured into the large wooden barrel to cover the chest（Fig. 15-4）.

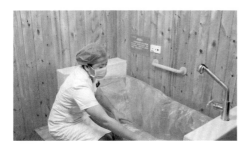

图 15-3　垫一次性泡浴袋

Fig. 15-3   Putting a disposable bath bag

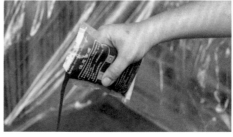

图 15-4　倒入药液

Fig. 15-4   Pouring liquid medicine into the large wooden barrel

②入浴。放入浴桶架，待药液温度在 40 ～ 45 ℃时，嘱患者取坐姿，将躯体四肢浸泡在药液中（图 15-5）。

② Balneation. A wooden barrel rack is put in the barrel and the patient is instructed to take the sitting position for soaking in the liquid medicine when the temperature of the liquid medicine is 40 ～ 45 ℃（Fig. 15-5）.

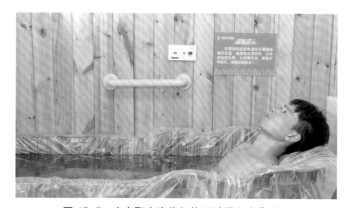

图 15-5　患者取坐姿将躯体四肢浸泡在药液中
Fig. 15-5　Soaking in the liquid medicine in a sitting position

③泡浴。嘱患者一边浸泡一边揉搓或按压全身或患部，促进血液循环，以利于药物吸收（图 15-6）。

③ Bath. The patient is instructed to rub or press the whole body or the affected part to promote blood circulation and facilitate drug absorption（Fig. 15-6）.

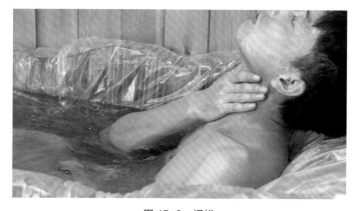

图 15-6　揉搓
Fig. 15-6　Rubbing

④泡浴后让患者用浴巾擦干全身，及时穿衣保暖。

④ The patient wipes the body with a towel after taking a bath and dresses warmly in time.

（4）整理患者衣物及操作物品。

（4）The doctor tidies up the patient's clothing and used materials.

（5）交代患者治疗后注意事项等。

（5）The doctor informs the patient of precautions after treatment.

（6）洗手并记录治疗情况。

（6）The doctor washes hands and makes a record about treatment.

六、疗程
VI　Course of treatment

每天1次，7天为1个疗程，根据患者病情适当增加疗程。

Once a day, 7 days as a course of treatment. Based on the patient's disease condition, increase the course of treatment properly.

七、注意事项
VII　Notes

（1）患者过度疲劳、过度饥饿、过度饱或精神高度紧张时不能操作。暴露治疗部位时，应注意保护患者隐私。

（1）It is prohibited for patients who suffer from excessive fatigue, excessive hunger, overeating or high mental stress. When the treatment area is exposed, the doctor should protect the patient's privacy and keep the patient warm.

（2）药浴全程陪护观察患者情况，提供温水或姜糖水，嘱患者少量多次饮用以补充水分，如觉疲劳或不适可到旁边座椅或按摩床上稍作休息。

（2）The doctor should observe the patient's condition during the medicated bath and provide warm freshwater or ginger syrup. Besides, the doctor should instruct the patient to drink a small amount of water. If the patient feels tired or discomfort，he/she can take a rest on the chair or massage table.

（3）药液温度要适中，不能过烫，以免烫伤。

（3）The temperature of the liquid medicine should be moderate to avoid scald.

（4）注意控制泡浴时间，每次 20～30 分钟为宜（视患者耐受情况可酌减）。年老体弱者泡浴时间不宜过长。

（4）Pay attention to the bath time which may last 20 to 30 minutes each time（it can be reduced depending on the patient's tolerance）. Moreover，the bath time for the elderly and the infirm should not be too long.

（5）患者泡浴时要避免受寒、吹风，泡浴完毕应立即拭干皮肤，注意保暖。

（5）The patient should avoid catching a cold when taking a bath. Moreover，the patient should immediately wipe off the water and keep warm after taking a bath.

（6）空腹及饭后 30 分钟内不宜泡浴。

（6）It is not advisable to take a bath on an empty stomach or within 30 minutes after a meal.

（7）泡浴后禁止剧烈运动或劳累。

（7）It is prohibited to do vigorous exercise after the bath.

八、意外情况及处理

Ⅷ　Accidents and handling methods

（1）晕泡。泡浴过程中如患者出现气短、面色苍白、出冷汗等症状，立即让患者出浴，取头低位平卧 10 分钟左右，亦可加服少量糖水；若出现严重至昏迷不醒者，立即行急救处理。

（1）Fainting. If the patient develops shortness of breath，pale complexion and cold sweat，this operation should be stopped immediately，and help the patient lie flat with head-down tilt for about 10 minutes and drink a small amount of sugar water. If the patient is unconscious，an emergency treatment should be performed immediately.

（2）烫伤、起水疱。如有烫伤，用生理盐水清洁创面并浸润无菌纱布湿敷创面直至疼痛明显减轻或消失后，外涂烧伤膏。皮肤若出现小水疱，可自行吸收，保持局部干燥及水疱皮肤的完整性即可；如水疱较大，可用无菌针头将水疱戳破，放出疱内渗液，每天用碘伏消毒，外涂烧伤膏，保持局部干燥及清洁，预防感染。

（2）Scalds and blisters. For scalds，the surface of the wound should be disinfected with physiological saline and compressed by wet sterile gauzes until the pain is greatly relieved or disappears，and then applied burn ointment. For small blisters，the skin will absorb the blisters fluid if the skin over the blisters is not open and kept dry. For large blisters，a sterile needle can be used to puncture them to release the fluid. The patient should disinfect it with iodophor and apply burn ointment to it. Besides，the patient should keep the skin dry and clean every day to prevent infection.

【附注】
【Notes】

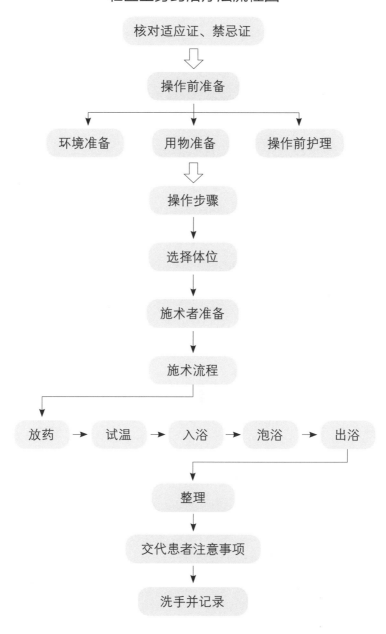

壮医全身药浴疗法流程图

The Flow Chart about Zhuang Medicine Whole Body Medicated Bath Therapy

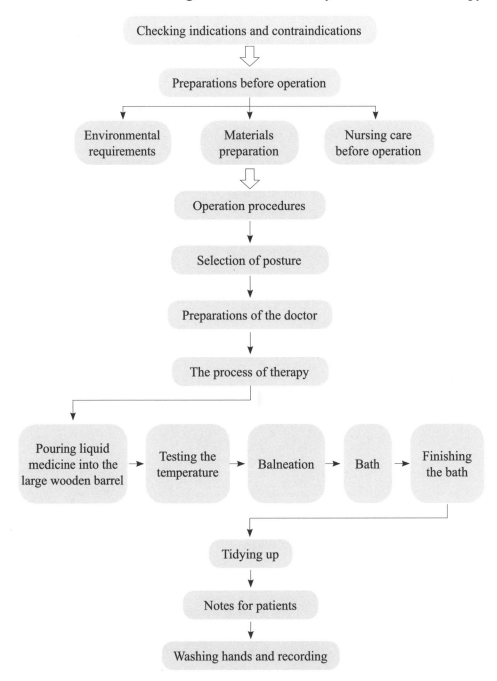

第十六章　壮医敷贴疗法
Chapter 16　Zhuang Medicine Application Therapy

壮医敷贴疗法是将壮药研成细粉后制成药饼，敷贴于人体某些部位或穴位，通过皮肤对药物的吸收，以治疗疾病的一种方法。

Zhuang medicine application therapy refers to a therapeutic method of sticking Zhuang medicinal cakes on the affected part or acupoints to let the skin absorb the medicine to treat the disease.

一、主要功效
Ⅰ　Main effects

祛风、湿、寒、痰、瘀等毒，散结，消肿，补虚强体，通调三道两路，调节气血平衡。

To dispel wind, dampness, cold, phlegm and blood stasis. To eliminate stagnation and swelling, restore vital energy, regulate three passages and two pathways, and the balance between qi and blood, etc.

二、适应证
Ⅱ　Indications

内科、外科、妇科、儿科、五官科等常见病、多发病均可使用本疗法治疗，常见适应证有楞涩（鼻炎）、奔唉（咳嗽）、奔墨（哮喘）、发旺（痹病）、麻邦（中风）、血压嗓（原发性高血压）、年闹诺（失眠）、胴尹（胃痛）、奔鹿（呕吐）、沙呃（呃逆）、核嘎尹（腰腿痛）、活邀尹（颈椎病）、旁巴尹（肩周炎）、骆芡（骨性关节炎）、林得叮相（跌打损伤）、京尹（痛经）、嘻缶（乳腺增生）、航靠谋（腮腺炎）、勒爷屙细（小儿泄泻）、勒爷唉疳（小儿疳积）、勒爷病卟哏（小儿厌食症）等。

This therapy can be used to treat the common diseases and frequently-occurring diseases of internal medicine, surgery, gynecology, pediatrics, ENT, etc. Its common indications include Lengse（rhinitis）, Ben'ai（cough）, Benmo（asthma）, Fawang（arthralgia disease）, Mabang（stroke）, Xueyasang（essential hypertension）, Niannaonuo（insomnia）, Dongyin（stomachache）, Benlu（vomiting）, Sha'e（hiccough）, Hegayin（lumbocrural pain）, Huoyaoyin（cervical spondylosis）, Pangbayin（scapulohumeral periarthritis）, Luoqian（osteoarthritis）, Lindedingxiang（traumatic injury）, Jingyin（dysmenorrhea）, Xifou（hyperplasia of mammary glands）, Hangkaomou（parotitis）, Leye'exi（infantile diarrhea）, Leyebengan（infantile malnutrition）, Leyebingbugen（infantile anorexia）, etc.

三、禁忌证
Ⅲ　Contraindications

（1）孕妇禁用。

（1）It is prohibited for pregnant women.

（2）皮肤过敏者、局部皮肤溃烂者禁用。

（2）It is prohibited for patients suffering from skin allergies and local skin ulcers.

（3）开放性创口或感染性病灶处禁用。

（3）It is prohibited for patients who have open wounds or infectious lesions.

四、操作前准备
Ⅳ　Preparations before operation

（1）环境要求。治疗室内清洁，安静，光线明亮，温度适宜，避免患者吹风受凉。

（1）Environmental requirements. The treatment room should be clean, quiet and well-lit. Besides，keep the treatment room at an ideal temperature to prevent the patient from catching a cold.

（2）用物准备。一次性无纺布穴位敷贴胶布贴、纱布、绷带、胶布、压板、药粉（图 16-1）、姜汁（或米醋、黄酒）、生理盐水、消毒棉签、一次性无菌手套、剪刀等。

（2）Materials preparation. Disposable non-woven acupoint application，gauzes，bandages，adhesive plasters，spatulas，medicinal powder（Fig. 16-1），ginger juice（or rice vinegar，rice wine），physiological saline，sterile cotton swabs，disposable sterile gloves，scissors，etc.

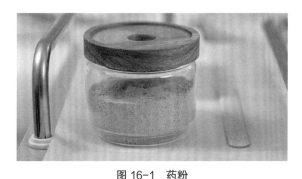

图 16-1　药粉
Fig. 16-1　Medicinal powder

（3）操作前护理。说明治疗的意义和注意事项，取得患者同意；对患者进行精神安慰与鼓励，消除患者的紧张、恐惧情绪，使患者能积极主动配合操作。

（3）Nursing care before operation. The nurse should explain the significance and notices of the treatment to obtain the patient's consent. Besides，the nurse should encourage the patient to overcome his/her nervousness and fear and enable the patient to cooperate with the doctor for a better operation.

五、操作步骤
V　Operation procedures

（1）体位选择。根据患者病情确定体位，常取坐位、俯卧位、仰卧位、侧卧位等，以患者舒适及便于施术者操作为宜，避免用强迫体位。

（1）Posture selection. Based on the state of the illness，the posture is selected. Sitting position，prone position，dorsal position or lateral-recumbent position is often selected to provide convenience for the patient and the doctor. The compulsive position should be avoided.

（2）部位选择。根据病证选取相应的治疗部位或穴位。

（2）Position selection. According to the disease patterns，the corresponding treatment area is selected.

（3）洗手，戴医用外科口罩、医用帽子和一次性无菌手套。

（3）The doctor should wash hands，then，wear a surgical mask，a medical cap and disposable sterile gloves.

（4）清洁。用生理盐水清洁施术部位的皮肤（图 16-2）。

（4）Cleaning. Clean the skin of treatment areas with physiological saline（Fig. 16-2）.

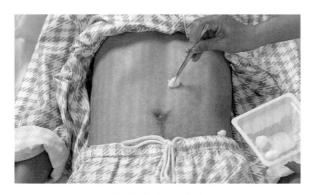

图 16-2　清洁皮肤
Fig. 16-2　Cleaning the skin

（5）施术流程。

（5）Operation procedures.

①调药。将药物粉末加适量姜汁（或米醋、黄酒）调和，干湿适中（图 16-3、图 16-4）。

①Blending the medicinal powder. The appropriate amount of medicinal powder is blended with ginger juice（or rice vinegar，rice wine）（Fig. 16-3，Fig. 16-4）.

②捏药饼。将药粉加工成圆饼（圆饼大小视治疗部位而定）（图 16-5、图

16-6）。

② Kneading the medicinal cakes. The medicinal powder is processed into round cakes（the size of the round cakes depends on the treatment areas）（Fig. 16-5, Fig. 16-6）.

③敷贴。将药饼贴在选定的部位或穴位上（图 16-7），用胶布固定。

③ Application. The medicinal cakes are sticked on the selected parts or acupoints（Fig. 16-7）and fixed with adhesive plasters.

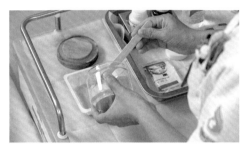

图 16-3　加入姜汁
Fig. 16-3　Adding ginger juice

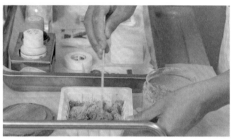

图 16-4　搅拌混合
Fig. 16-4　Stirring and blending

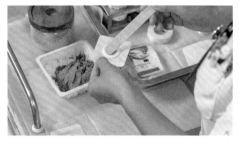

图 16-5　制药饼
Fig. 16-5　Making the medicinal cakes

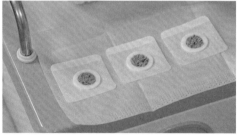

图 16-6　制成待用
Fig. 16-6　For later use

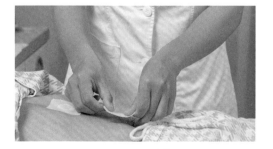

图 16-7　贴药
Fig. 16-7　Sticking medicinal cakes

（6）整理患者衣物及操作物品。

（6）The doctor tidies up the patient's clothing and used materials.

（7）交代患者治疗后注意事项等。

（7）The doctor informs the patient of precautions after treatment.

（8）洗手并记录治疗情况。

（8）The doctor washes hands and makes a record about treatment.

六、疗程
Ⅵ　Course of treatment

一般每天 1 次，病情症状严重者可每天 2 次，14 天为 1 个疗程。

Once a day in general，twice a day for severe symptoms，14 days as a course of treatment.

七、注意事项
Ⅶ　Notes

（1）患者过度饥饿、过度饱或精神高度紧张时不能操作。暴露治疗部位时，应注意保护患者隐私及保暖。

（1）It is prohibited for patients who suffer from excessive hunger，overeating or high mental stress. When treatment areas are exposed，the doctor should protect the patient's privacy and keep the patient warm.

（2）敷贴局部可能会有微红、轻度瘙痒、色素沉着等现象，均为正常反应。

（2）There may be redness，mild itching and pigmentation on treatment areas，which is normal.

（3）嘱患者严格遵循敷贴时间，儿童不宜超过 1 小时，成人 2～4 小时，不宜擅自延长时间。

（3）The patient is instructed to strictly follow the application time which should not exceed 1 hour for children and 2 to 4 hours for adults. It is not advisable to extend the application time.

（4）必须交代患者注意敷贴部位的感觉，如敷贴后皮肤出现瘙痒难耐、灼热、疼痛等感觉时，应立即取下药膏，并禁止抓挠，注意保持清洁，不宜擅自涂抹别的药物，一般轻症可自愈。若皮肤出现红肿、水疱、破溃等严重反应，需及时到医院就诊。

（4）The doctor should instruct the patient to pay attention to the feeling about the treated areas. If there is itching, burning, and painful sensation on the skin, the medicinal cakes should be removed immediately. Besides, do not scratch, keep the skin clean. It is not advisable to apply other ointments because mild symptoms can be self-cure. If the skin has severe reactions such as redness, swellings, blisters, and ulcerations, it is necessary to go to the hospital in time.

（5）根据自身病情，患者治疗后在饮食上应注意忌口（如忌食生冷、油腻、发物等），以清淡饮食为主。

（5）According to the disease condition, the patient should avoid eating cold dishes, oily food and stimulating food as well as should eat a bland diet after treatment.

八、意外情况及处理
Ⅷ　Accidents and handling methods

如有过敏反应，应立即停止敷贴，若症状轻微无须特别治疗，必要时给予抗过敏药物治疗。

If there is an allergic reaction, the application should be stopped immediately. If the symptoms are mild, special treatment is not required. If the symptoms are severe, anti-allergic drug treatment is required.

【附注】
【Notes】

常用敷贴药物制备
Preparation of Commonly Used Herbs for Application Therapy

（1）材料制作。根据不同病证选用方剂，取干品饮片打粉备用。

（1）Materials preparation. Different prescriptions are selected according to different disease patterns, and then decoction pieces are ground into powder for later use.

如通痹膏药物：黑老虎、飞龙掌血、干姜、桂枝、制川乌、制附子、羌活、大血藤、宽筋藤、丁香、花椒等。

Herbs for treating arthralgia：Heilaohu（Radix et Caulis Kadsurae Coccineae）, Feilongzhangxue（Radix Toddaliae Asiaticae）, Ganjiang（Rhizoma Zingiberis）, Guizhi（Ramulus Cinnamomi）, Zhichuanwu（Radix Aconiti Preparata）, Zhifuzi（Radix Aconiti Lateralis Preparata）, Qianghuo（Rhizoma et Radix Notopterygii）, Daxueteng（Caulis Sargentodoxae）, Kuanjinteng（Caulis Tinosporae Sinensis）, Dingxiang（Flos Caryophylli）, Huajiao（Pericarpium Zanthoxyli）, etc.

（2）调和药液制备。根据不同病证选用姜汁、米醋、黄酒等。

（2）Preparation of liquid medicine. Ginger juice, rice vinegar or rice wine is selected according to the disease patterns.

壮医敷贴疗法流程图

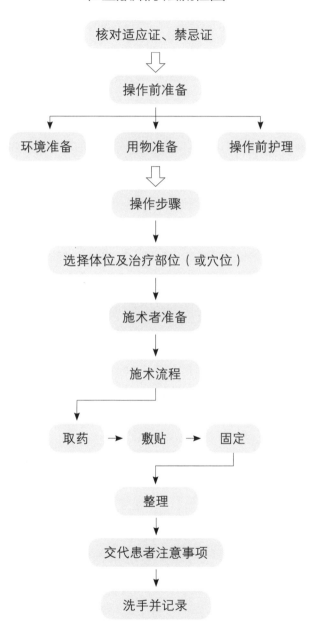

The Flow Chart about Zhuang Medicine Application Therapy

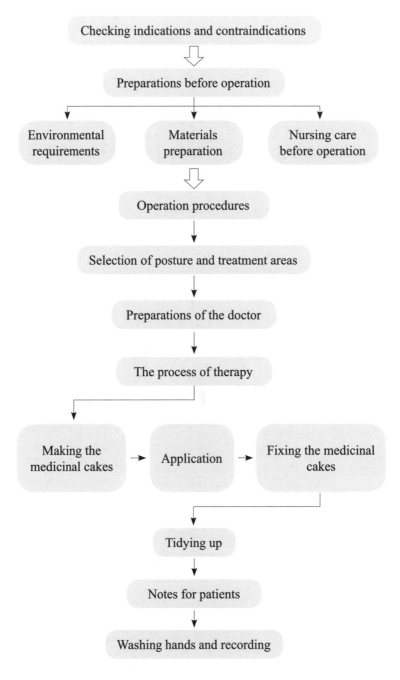

第十七章 壮医滚蛋疗法
Chapter 17 Zhuang Medicine Egg-Rolling Therapy

壮医滚蛋疗法是在壮医理论指导下，用新鲜生蛋（冷滚法）或经过加工的熟蛋（热滚法）在身体有关部位来回滚动，以预防或治疗疾病的一种方法。

Zhuang medicine egg-rolling therapy refers to a therapeutic method of rolling back and forth on relevant parts of the body with fresh raw eggs（cold rolling manipulation）or boiled eggs（hot rolling manipulation）to prevent or treat diseases under the guidance of Zhuang medical theory.

一、主要功效
I Main effects

祛风、湿、痧、瘴、热、寒、痰、瘀等毒，消肿，散结，止痛，通调三道两路，调节气血平衡。

To dispel wind, dampness, pathogen, miasma, fever, cold, phlegm and blood stasis. To eliminate swelling, stagnation and pain. To regulate three passages and two pathways, and the balance between qi and blood.

二、适应证
II Indications

内科、外科、妇科、儿科、皮肤科等常见病、多发病均可使用本疗法治疗，常见适应证有得凉（感冒、上呼吸道感染）、奔唉（咳嗽）、发旺（痹病）、林得叮相（跌打损伤）、朗尹（肌肉关节疼痛）等。

This therapy can be used to treat the common diseases and frequently-occurring diseases of internal medicine, surgery, gynecology, pediatrics, dermatology, etc. Its common indications include Deliang（cold，upper respiratory tract infection）, Benài（cough）, Fawang（arthralgia disease）, Lindedingxiang（traumatic injury）, Langyin（muscle and joint pain）, etc.

三、禁忌证
Ⅲ　Contraindications

（1）开放性创口或感染性病灶处禁用。

（1）It is prohibited for patients who have open wounds or infectious lesions.

（2）皮肤过敏者、局部皮肤溃烂者禁用。

（2）It is prohibited for patients who suffer from skin allergies and local skin ulcers.

四、操作前准备
Ⅳ　Preparations before operation

（1）环境要求。治疗室内清洁，安静，光线明亮，温度适宜，避免患者吹风受凉。

（1）Environmental requirements. The treatment room should be clean，quiet and well-lit. Besides，keep the treatment room at an ideal temperature to prevent the patient from catching a cold.

（2）用物准备。

（2）Materials preparation.

①准备鸡蛋或鸭蛋2个。一般选用鸡蛋，以新鲜为佳。

① 2 hen's eggs or 2 duck's eggs should be prepared. Fresh hen's eggs are generally used.

②药物。根据患者病情选择相应药物（如感冒选用生姜20 g，艾叶30 g，葱白10 g等；风湿病选用杜仲15 g，羌活15 g，独活10 g，桑枝15 g等；跌打损伤选用桃仁10 g，红花10 g，迎春花15 g，天门冬20 g等；消化不良选用山楂15 g，鸡内金15 g，神曲15 g等）。

② Medicinal materials. Corresponding medicinal materials are chosen by the doctor according to the patient's disease condition. For example, medicinal materials to treat cold include Shengjiang（Rhizoma Zingiberis Recens）20 g, Aiye（Folium Artemisiae Argyi）30 g, Congbai（Bulbus Allii Fistulosi）10 g, etc. Medicinal materials to treat rheumatism include Duzhong（Cortex Eucommiae）15 g, Qianghuo（Rhizoma et Radix Notopterygii）15 g, Duhuo（Radix Angelicae Pubescentis）10 g, Sangzhi（Ramulus Mori）15 g, etc. Medicinal materials to treat traumatic injury include Taoren（Semen Persicae）10 g, Honghua（Flos Carthami）10 g, Yingchunhua（Folium et Flos Jasmini Nudiflori）15 g, Tianmendong（Radix Asparagi）20 g, etc. Medicinal materials to treat indigestion include Shanzha（Fructus Crataegi）15 g, Jineijin（Endothelium Corneum Gigeriae Galli）15 g, Shenqu（Massa Medicata Fermentata）15 g, etc.

③一次性无菌手套、医用纱布。

③ Disposable sterile gloves and medical gauzes.

（3）操作前护理。核对患者信息及治疗方案等，说明治疗的意义和注意事项，取得患者同意；对患者进行精神安慰与鼓励，消除患者的紧张、恐惧情绪，使患者能积极主动配合操作。

（3）Nursing care before operation. The nurse should check the patient's information and treatment plan and explain the significance and notices of the treatment to obtain the patient's consent. Besides, the nurse should encourage the patient to overcome his/her nervousness and fear and enable the patient to cooperate with the doctor for a better operation.

五、操作步骤
V Operation procedures

（1）体位选择。根据患者病情确定体位，常取坐位、俯卧位、仰卧位、侧卧位等，以患者舒适及便于施术者操作为宜，避免用强迫体位。

（1）Posture selection. Based on the state of the illness, the posture is selected. Sitting position, prone position, dorsal position or lateral recumbent position is often selected to provide convenience for the patient and the doctor. The compulsive position should be avoided.

（2）部位选择。根据病证选取适当的治疗部位。

（2）Position selection. According to the disease patterns，the corresponding treatment area is selected.

（3）洗手，戴医用外科口罩、医用帽子和一次性无菌手套。

（3）The doctor should wash hands，then，wear a surgical mask，a medical cap and disposable sterile gloves.

（4）清洁。用生理盐水清洁施术部位表面皮肤。

（4）Cleaning. Clean the skin of treatment areas with physiological saline.

（5）施术流程。

（5）Operation procedures.

①煮蛋。往准备好的药物中加入 750 ～ 1000 mL 水（图 17-1），取蛋加入其中与药物同煮（图 17-2）。

① Boiling eggs. The doctor adds 750 to 1000 mL of water into the prepared medicinal materials in a pot（Fig. 17-1），and then puts eggs into it to boil（Fig. 17-2）.

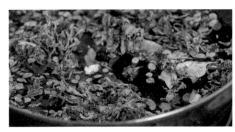

图 17-1　煮药
Fig. 17-1　Decocting medicinal materials and eggs

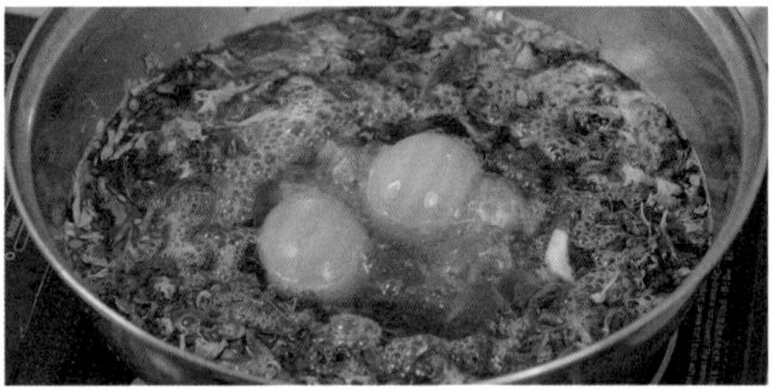

图 17-2　放蛋
Fig. 17-2　Putting eggs in the water

②剥蛋。蛋煮熟后剥壳（图 17-3），浸于药液中保温备用（图 17-4）。

② Peeling eggs. The doctor should peel eggs after they are boiled（Fig. 17-3），and then soak them in the liquid medicine to keep them warm for later use（Fig. 17-4）.

③滚蛋。将煮熟的蛋从保温的药液中取出，趁热在患者头部、额部、颈部、

胸部、背部、四肢、手掌心、脚底心依次反复滚动热熨（图 17-5、图 17-6、图 17-7），至患者微微汗出而止。蛋凉后，可再放入药液中加热，2 个蛋轮流使用。若采用冷滚法则无须加热。

③ Rolling eggs. The doctor takes the boiled eggs out of warm liquid medicine，and then rolls warm eggs repeatedly to iron the head，forehead，neck，chest，back，limbs，palms，and soles of the feet（Fig. 17-5，Fig.17-6，Fig. 17-7）until the patient slightly sweats. When eggs get cold，they can be put into the liquid medicine for heating. Moreover，two eggs can be used in turn. Cold rolling manipulation does not require heating.

（6）施术后处理。用医用纱布清洁施术部位皮肤（图 17-8），将用过的蛋放入黄色废物袋。

（6）Postoperative treatment. The doctor cleans the skin with medical gauzes（Fig. 17-8）and places the used eggs into a yellow waste bag.

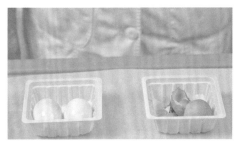

图 17-3　剥蛋

Fig. 17-3　Peeling eggs

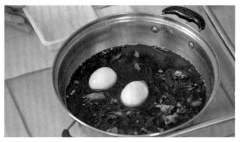

图 17-4　鸡蛋保温

Fig. 17-4　Eggs' heat preservation

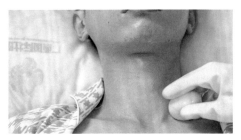

图 17-5　在颈部滚动

Fig. 17-5　Rolling on the neck

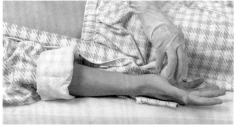

图 17-6　在掌心滚动

Fig. 17-6　Rolling on the palm

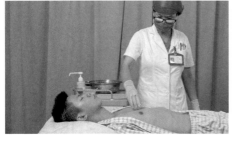

图 17-7　在胸部滚动

Fig. 17-7　Rolling on the chest

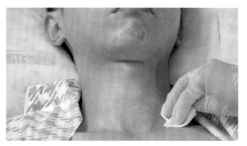

图 17-8　施术后清洁

Fig. 17-8　Postoperative clean

（7）整理患者衣物及操作物品。

（7）The doctor tidies up the patient's clothing and used materials.

（8）交代患者治疗后注意事项等。

（8）The doctor informs the patient of precautions after treatment.

（9）洗手并记录治疗情况。

（9）The doctor washes hands and makes a record about treatment.

六、疗程
Ⅵ　Course of treatment

每次 20 ～ 30 分钟，每天 1 ～ 2 次，5 ～ 7 天为 1 个疗程。

20 to 30 minutes each time，once or twice a day，5 to 7 days as a course of treatment.

七、注意事项
Ⅶ　Notes

（1）患者过度饥饿、过度饱或精神高度紧张时不能操作。暴露治疗部位时，应注意保护患者隐私及保暖。

（1）It is prohibited for patients who suffer from excessive hunger，overeating or high mental stress. When treatment areas are exposed，the doctor should protect the patient's privacy and keep the patient warm.

（2）应用壮医滚蛋疗法时，如结合推拿疗法效果更好。

（2）When applying Zhuang medicine egg-rolling therapy，the doctor may combine it with massage，which will have a better effect.

（3）滚蛋要有侧重点，头痛则在头部滚的时间长些，腹痛则在腹部滚的时间长些，腰痛则在腰部滚的时间长些。

（3）Egg-rolling therapy has points of focus. The time of rolling on the head should be longer than that on other parts for treating headache. The time of rolling on the abdomen should be longer than that on other parts for treating abdominal pain. The time of rolling on the waist should be longer than that on other parts for treating low back pain.

（4）蛋的温度以患者耐受为宜，避免烫伤。

（4）The temperature of the eggs should be tolerated by the patient to avoid scald.

（5）用来做滚蛋的蛋不宜再食用，以免将排出的毒素再摄入体内。

（5）The patient should not eat these eggs so as not to re-intake the toxin into the body.

八、意外情况及处理
Ⅷ　Accidents and handling methods

如有烫伤，用生理盐水清洁创面并浸润无菌纱布湿敷创面直至疼痛明显减轻或消失后，外涂烧伤膏。如起小水疱，皮肤可自行吸收，保持局部干燥及水疱皮肤的完整性即可；如水疱较大，可用无菌针头将水疱戳破，放出疱内渗液，每天用碘伏消毒，外涂烧伤膏，保持局部干燥及清洁，预防感染。

For scalds，the surface of the wound should be disinfected with physiological saline and compressed by wet sterile gauzes until the pain is greatly relieved or disappears，and then applied burn ointment. For small blisters，the skin will absorb the blisters fluid if the skin over the blisters is not open and kept dry. For large blisters，a sterile needle can be used to puncture them to release the fluid. The patient should disinfect it with iodophor and apply burn ointment to it. Besides，the patient should keep the skin dry and clean every day to prevent infection.

【附注】
【Notes】

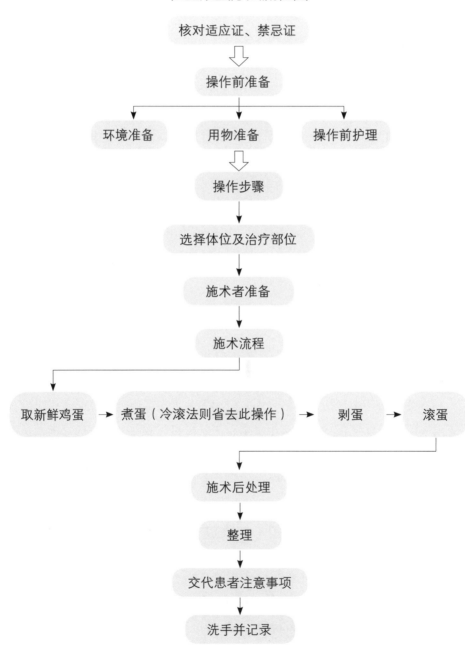

壮医滚蛋疗法流程图

The Flow Chart about Zhuang Medicine Egg-Rolling Therapy

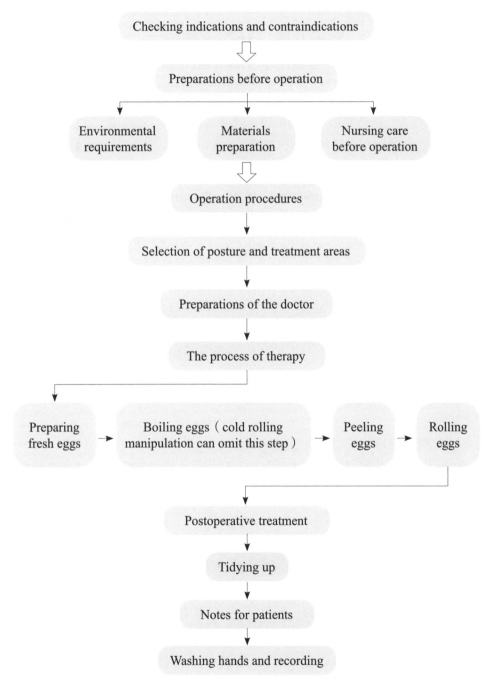

第十八章 壮医水蛭疗法
Chapter 18 Zhuang Medicine Leech Therapy

壮医水蛭疗法是利用饥饿的活体水蛭对人体体表道路网结（穴位或痛点）进行吸治，吸拔局部瘀滞的气血，同时释放水蛭素入人体，从而疏通三道两路，维持人体天、地、人三气同步，调节气血平衡，以治疗疾病的一种方法。

Zhuang medicine leech therapy refers to a therapeutic method of using hungry leeches to suck local stagnant qi and blood on the meridian（acupoints or pain points）and release hirudin into the human body to regulate three passages and two pathways and the balance between qi and blood as well as maintain three-qi harmony.

一、主要功效
I Main effects

用于风、寒、湿、痰、瘀等毒所导致三道两路不通、机体平衡失调而引起的病证。

To dispel wind，cold，dampness，phlegm，blood stasis，etc. These disease patterns can cause the obstruction of three passages and two pathways as well as the imbalance between qi and blood.

二、适应证
II Indications

内科、外科、妇科、儿科、五官科、皮肤科等常见病、多发病均可使用本疗法治疗，常见适应证有喯呗啷（带状疱疹、带状疱疹后遗神经痛）、能啥累（瘙痒、湿疹）、痂怀（银屑病）、泵栾（脱发）、邦呷（脑梗死后遗症）、哪呷（面瘫）、巧尹（头痛）、年闹诺（失眠）、三叉神经痛、楞瑟（鼻炎）、阿闷（胸痹）、静脉曲张、脉管炎、发旺（痹病）、隆芡（痛风）、令扎（强直性脊柱炎）、能嘎累（臁疮）、旁巴尹（肩周炎）、皮下脂肪瘤、嘻缶（乳腺增生）、手术后皮瓣静脉瘀血、呗哝（痈疮肿痛）、腊胴尹（腹痛）、奔浮（水肿）、幽堆（前列腺炎）、约京乱（月经不调）、子宫唪北（子宫肌瘤）、卟很裆（不孕不育）等。

This therapy can be used to treat the common diseases and frequently-occurring diseases of internal medicine，surgery，gynecology，pediatrics，ENT，dermatology，etc. Its common indications include Benbeilang（shingles，postherpetic neuralgia），Nenghanlei（pruritus，eczema），Jiahuai（psoriasis），Bengluan（alopecia），Bangxia（sequela of cerebral infarction），Naxia（facial paralysis），Qiaoyin（headache），Niannaonuo（insomnia），trigeminal neuralgia，Lengse（rhinitis），Amen（thoracic obstruction），varix，angiitis，Fawang（arthralgia disease），Longqian（gout），Lingzha（ankylosing spondylitis），Nenggalei（ecthyma），Pangbayin（scapulohumeral periarthritis），lipoma，Xifou（hyperplasia of mammary glands），postoperative flap venous congestion，Beinong（ulcerative carbuncle，swelling and pain），Ladongyin（abdominal pain），Benfu（edema），Youdui（prostatitis），Yuejingluan（irregular menstruation），Zigongbenbei（hysteromyoma），Buhendang（infertility），etc.

三、禁忌证
Ⅲ　Contraindications

（1）自发出血性疾病患者、凝血功能障碍者、出血性脑血管疾病（急性期）患者禁用。

（1）It is prohibited for patients who suffer from spontaneous bleeding disorders，coagulation disorders or hemorrhagic cerebrovascular diseases（acute phase）.

（2）具急性心肌梗死、高血压危象、呼吸衰竭、严重肝病及肝功能衰竭、急慢性肾衰竭、肿瘤晚期等引起恶病质状态者禁用。

（2）It is prohibited for patients who suffer from acute myocardial infarction，hypertensive crisis，respiratory failure，severe liver disease and liver failure，acute and chronic renal failure，or advanced tumor，etc.

（3）月经量多或处于崩漏状态者、孕期及产后（或小产后）1个月内者禁用。

（3）It is prohibited for patients who suffer from hypermenorrhea，metrorrhagia，or who are pregnant and postpartum（miscarriage）within 1 month.

（4）晕针或晕血者，对痛觉高度敏感者，精神病患者，精神高度紧张、狂躁不安、抽搐不能合作者禁用。

（4）It is prohibited for patients who suffer from fainting during acupuncture and blood phobia. Besides，it is prohibited for patients who are highly sensitive to pain，psychotic，high mental stress，manic，anxious，or spasmodic.

（5）对水蛭恐惧者、糖尿病合并并发症者、大量饮酒者、皮肤严重过敏者、长期服用抗凝药物者慎用。

（5）It should be used cautiously for patients suffering from fear of leeches，diabetes complications，heavy drinking and severe skin allergies. Besides，patients taking anticoagulant drugs for a long time also needs to use it cautiously.

四、操作前准备
Ⅳ　Preparations before operation

（1）环境要求。治疗室内清洁，安静，光线明亮，温度适宜，避免患者吹风受凉。

（1）Environmental requirements. The treatment room should be clean，quiet and well-lit. Besides，keep the treatment room at an ideal temperature to prevent the patient from catching a cold.

（2）用物准备。经过净化并检验合格的医用水蛭、无齿镊子、无菌干棉球、医用棉签、医用纱布、无菌小方纱、一次性无菌手套、注射器针头、医用胶布、一次性换药碗、75%酒精、生理盐水、止血粉。

（2）Materials preparation. Purified and qualified medical leeches，smooth forceps，sterile dry cotton balls，medical cotton swabs，medical gauzes，sterile small gauzes，disposable sterile gloves，syringe needles，medical adhesive plasters，disposable dressing bowls，75% alcohol，physiological saline，hemostatic powder.

（3）操作前护理。核对患者信息及治疗方案等，说明治疗的意义和注意事项，取得患者同意；对患者进行精神安慰与鼓励，消除患者的紧张、恐惧情绪，使患者能积极主动配合操作。

（3）Nursing care before operation. The nurse should check the patient's information and treatment plan and explain the significance and notices of the treatment to obtain the patient's consent. Besides，the nurse should encourage the patient to overcome his/her nervousness and fear and enable the patient to cooperate with the doctor for a better operation.

五、操作步骤
V　Operation procedures

（1）体位选择。根据患者病情确定体位，常取坐位、俯卧位、仰卧位、侧卧位等，以患者舒适及便于施术者操作为宜，避免用强迫体位。

（1）Posture selection. Based on the state of the illness，the posture is selected. Sitting position，prone position，dorsal position or lateral recumbent position is often selected to provide convenience for the patient and the doctor. The compulsive position should be avoided.

（2）部位选择。根据病证选取相应的治疗部位，部位的选择侧重在患部、疼痛点或相应穴位，避开浅表大血管。

（2）Position selection. The corresponding treatment areas are selected according to the disease patterns. Besides，treatment areas should be affected parts，pain points or corresponding acupuncture points and superficial large blood vessels should be avoided.

（3）洗手，戴医用外科口罩、医用帽子和一次性无菌手套。

（3）The doctor should wash hands，then，wear a surgical mask，a medical cap and disposable sterile gloves.

（4）消毒。用75%酒精消毒施术部位（图18-1），待干后，再用生理盐水去除消毒部位酒精异味。

（4）Disinfection. The doctor disinfects treatment areas with 75% alcohol（Fig. 18-1）, lets it dry, and then uses physiological saline to eliminate the odor of alcohol on treatment areas.

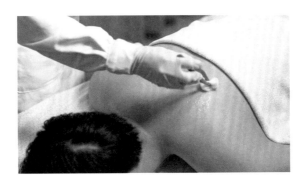

图 18-1　消毒施术部位
Fig. 18-1　Disinfection of treatment areas

（5）施术流程。

（5）Operation procedures.

①醒蛭。将生理盐水注入装水蛭的瓶管轻缓摇晃以清洗水蛭（图18-2），之后把水蛭放在一次性换药碗内待用（图18-3）。

① Washing leeches. The doctor fills the bottle with physiological saline, shakes it gently to wash leeches（Fig. 18-2）, then puts leeches in a disposable dressing bowl for later use（Fig. 18-3）.

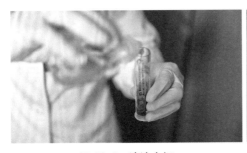

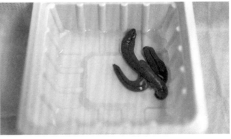

图 18-2　清洗水蛭
Fig. 18-2　Washing leeches

图 18-3　待用准备
Fig. 18-3　For later use

②定位。确定水蛭吸治的部位，做好标记。

② Positioning of treatment areas. The doctor identifies treatment areas where leeches will suck and marks them.

③吸治。用无齿镊子夹取水蛭（图18-4），用无菌小方纱包住水蛭后端，引导水蛭头部吸盘对准治疗部位（图18-5），稍作停留。若治疗部位的皮肤较厚或水蛭长时间未叮咬，可用注射器针头行局部刺血（图18-6）后再引导水蛭头部吸盘对准治疗部位使其叮吸（图18-7）。待水蛭叮吸固定后摊开纱布隔离水蛭与周围皮肤（图18-8），施术者全程监护。

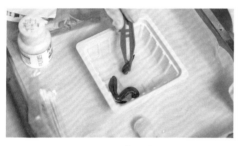

图 18-4　夹取水蛭

Fig. 18-4　Clamping the leech

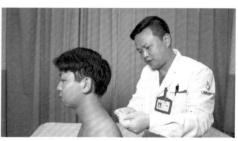

图 18-5　对准患部

Fig. 18-5　Aligning with the treatment areas

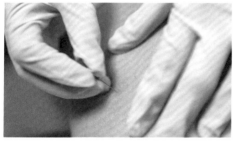

图 18-6　局部刺血

Fig. 18-6　Local blood-letting

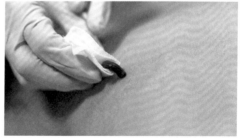

图 18-7　叮吸

Fig. 18-7　Sucting

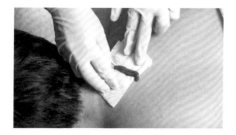

图 18-8　摊开纱布隔离

Fig. 18-8　Spreading out the gauze for isolation

③ Suck. The doctor uses smooth forceps to clamp the leech（Fig. 18-4）and wraps the rear end of the leech with a sterile small gauze. Then，the doctor makes the sucker of the leech align with the treatment areas（Fig. 18-5）and stops for a while. If the skin of the treatment areas is thick or the leech has not bitten for a long time，the doctor can puncture the treatment areas with the syringe needle（Fig. 18-6），and then make the sucker of the leech align with the treatment areas to make it bite（Fig. 18-7）. After the leech bites treatment areas，the doctor can spread out the gauze to isolate the leech from the surrounding skin（Fig. 18-8），and then monitor the whole process.

④取蛭。水蛭吸血饱食后会自动脱落，用无齿镊子将其钳至一次性换药碗内。吸治时间一般为 0.5 ～ 1 小时，如超过 1 小时水蛭仍不脱落，可使用医用棉签蘸 75％酒精涂抹水蛭吸盘（图 18-9），使水蛭自动脱落至换药碗内。

④ Taking the leech. The leech will fall off automatically after sucking enough blood，therefore，the doctor needs to use smooth forceps to put it into a disposable dressing bowl. In general，the suction time is about 0.5 to 1 hour. If the leech does not fall off after more than 1 hour，the doctor can use medical cotton swabs dipping 75% alcohol to apply to the sucker of the leech（Fig. 18-9），thus，the leech will automatically fall off into the dressing bowl.

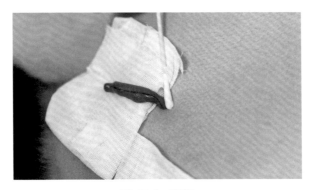

图 18-9　取蛭
Fig. 18-9　Taking the leech

⑤术毕，常规消毒治疗部位。

⑤ The doctor routinely disinfects treated areas after the operation.

⑥止血。用无菌干棉球按压吸治口 15 分钟，然后加无菌小方纱加压包扎后固定（图 18-10）；若出血无法止住，可在吸治口外敷止血粉后再包扎。

⑥ Stopping the bleeding. The doctor presses treated areas with a sterile dry cotton ball for 15 minutes, and then uses a sterile small square gauze to bind up and fix it（Fig. 18-10）. If the bleeding cannot be stopped, the doctor can apply hemostatic powder to treated areas before binding up.

（6）施术后处理。直接用 75％酒精浸泡水蛭令其死亡后做医疗垃圾处理（图 18-11）。吸治后的水蛭不可重复使用。

（6）Postoperative treatment. The doctor can immerse the leech directly with 75% alcohol to make it die, and then dispose of it（Fig. 18-11）. The used leeches are not recyclable.

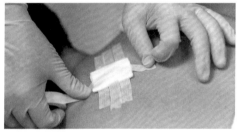 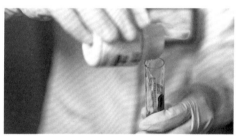

图 18-10　包扎伤口　　　　　　　　图 18-11　处理水蛭
Fig. 18-10　Binding up the wound　　　Fig. 18-11　Disposal of the leech

（7）整理患者衣物及操作物品。

（7）The doctor tidies up the patient's clothing and used materials.

（8）交代患者治疗后注意事项等。

（8）The doctor informs the patient of precautions after treatment.

（9）洗手并记录治疗情况。

（9）The doctor washes hands and makes a record about treatment.

六、疗程

Ⅵ Course of treatment

每周1～2次，每次水蛭吸血时间为0.5～1小时，连续治疗2周为1个疗程。

Once or twice a week. The sucking time of the leech is 0.5 to 1 hour each time and continuous treatment for 2 weeks is a course of treatment.

七、注意事项

Ⅶ Notes

（1）首次接受治疗者的水蛭用量不宜超过3条，之后重复治疗时水蛭用量不超过6条。

（1）The number of leeches should not exceed 3 for the first treatment and the number of leeches should not exceed 6 for repeated treatment.

（2）第二个疗程开始，可根据患者病情的变化，重新选择施术部位。如上一个疗程吸治口尚未愈合，可在吸治口附近选取新的部位，不宜重复在同一部位吸治。

（2）At the beginning of the second course of treatment，the doctor can reselect treatment areas according to the change of the disease condition. If the wound of the last course of treatment has not healed，a new part can be selected near the wound. It is not advisable to suck repeatedly at the same part.

（3）治疗前应与患者交代可能会出现色素沉着或留疤风险。对颜面部进行治疗前，建议先在患者身体其他部位施术，如无疤痕形成再治疗。

（3）The risk of pigmentation or scarring should be explained to the patient before treatment. The doctor should perform a trial on other parts of the body before facial treatment. If no scar occurs on other parts，the doctor can perform an operation on the face.

（4）静脉曲张、脉管炎等血管性疾病患者应注意做相关检查排除血栓形成及堵塞，并评估其风险和做好提示及告知。

（4）Vascular diseases including varicose veins and vasculitis should be checked by the doctor to exclude thrombosis and blockage. Besides，the doctor should assess risks and inform the patient.

（5）患者过度饥饿、过度饱或精神高度紧张时不能操作。暴露治疗部位时，应注意保护患者隐私及保暖。

（5）It is prohibited for patients who suffer from excessive hunger，overeating or high mental stress. When treatment areas are exposed，the doctor should protect the patient's privacy and keep the patient warm.

（6）治疗过程中宜让患者多饮温开水。

（6）It is advisable for the patient to drink warm water during the treatment.

（7）低血压或精神紧张者需监测血压。

（7）The doctor should monitor the blood pressure of patients who suffer from hypotension or nervousness.

（8）在头部、面部等部位施治时注意防止水蛭爬入口腔、鼻腔和耳朵等。

（8）Pay attention to preventing leeches from crawling into the patient's mouth，nose，ears，etc.

（9）高血压患者在治疗结束后应观察 30 分钟方可离开。

（9）Patients who suffer from hypertension should be observed for 30 minutes after treatment before they are allowed to leave.

（10）吸治口如出现血液渗出纱布现象，需重新加压包扎；或在吸治口外敷止血粉后再包扎。

（10）If the blood oozes out of the gauze from the wound，the doctor can use pressure bandaging. Besides，the doctor can apply hemostatic powder on the wound before bandaging.

（11）治疗后 24 小时内吸治口不可沾水。

（11）Treated areas should not get wet within 24 hours after treatment.

（12）所有治疗过程中使用过的物品应严格按照消毒隔离技术规范处理。

（12）All used materials should be handled in accordance with the standardized treatment of disinfection and isolation.

八、意外情况及处理

VIII Accidents and handling methods

（1）过敏。应立即停止吸治，若症状轻微者无须特别治疗，必要时给予抗过敏药物治疗。

（1）Allergies. Suck should be stopped immediately. If the symptoms are mild，no special treatment is required. If the symptoms are severe，anti-allergic drug treatment is required.

（2）感染。伤口如出现感染，及时就医。

（2）Infection. If the wound becomes infected，the patient should go to the hospital immediately.

（3）瘙痒。轻者用艾条灸熏瘙痒处，必要时及时就医。

（3）Itching. If the symptoms are mild，the patient can perform moxibustion on the itching area. If the symptoms are severe，the patient should go to the hospital immediately.

【附注】
【Notes】

壮医水蛭疗法流程图

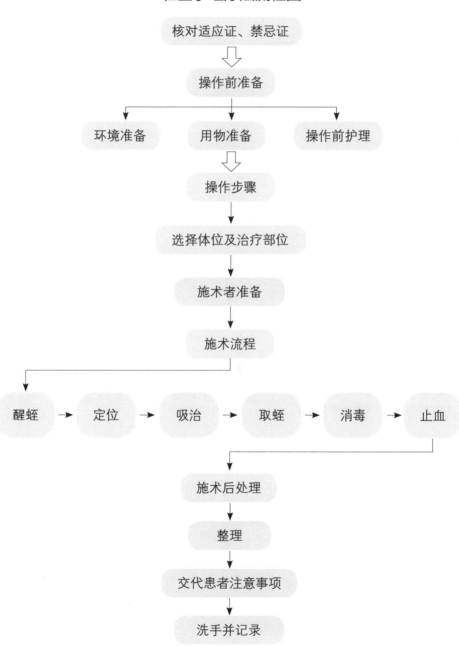

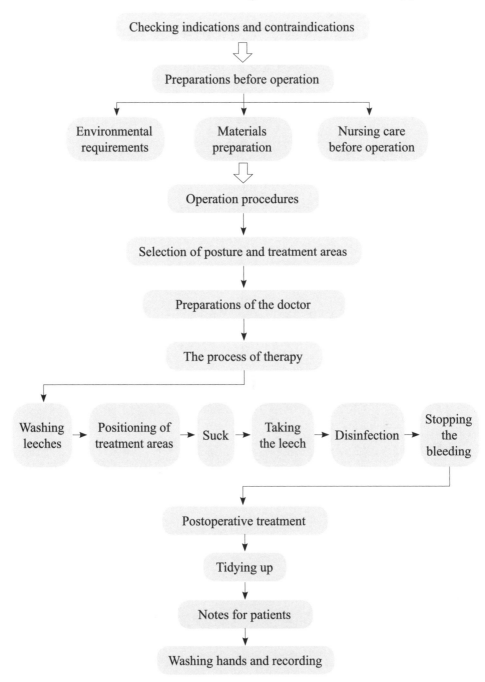

The Flow Chart about Zhuang Medicine Leech Therapy

参考文献

［1］陈攀，白露．壮医药线点灸手法概述［J］．亚太传统医药，2017，13（13）：15-16.

［2］樊鹤莹．彝医"滚蛋"疗法治疗小儿外感发热1566例临床研究［J］．中国民族医药杂志，2015，21（8）：18-19.

［3］何晓微，张云，黄欣．壮医药物竹罐疗法的临床应用概述［J］．中国民族医药杂志，2015，21（12）：11-12.

［4］黄汉儒．中国壮医学［M］．南宁：广西民族出版社，2000.

［5］黄瑾明，黄汉儒，黄鼎坚．壮医药线点灸疗法［M］．南宁：广西人民出版社，1986.

［6］黄瑾明，秦祖杰，宋宁，等．壮医脐环穴的历史渊源、理论基础与临床研究［J］．亚太传统医药，2019，15（10）：43-45.

［7］黄瑾明，宋宁，黄凯．中国壮医针灸学［M］．南宁：广西民族出版社，2010.

［8］黄贤忠．壮医针挑疗法（第2版）［M］．南宁：广西科学技术出版社，2000.

［9］黄艳宁．老壮医罗家安针挑疗法简介［J］．内蒙古中医药，1990（3）：20.

［10］蒋桂江，李凤珍，龙朝阳，等．壮医敷贴疗法文献记载及应用概况［J］．中国民族医药杂志，2016（3）：36-37.

［11］林辰，陈攀，黎玉宣．中国壮医外治学［M］．南宁：广西科学技术出版社，2015.

［12］林辰，吕琳．壮医外治学［M］．北京：中国中医药出版社，2017.

［13］吕琳，陈永红．壮医刺血疗法技术操作规范与应用研究［M］．南宁：广西科学技术出版社，2007.

［14］吕琳，韦金育，曾振东．壮医药线点灸疗法技术操作规范与应用研究［M］．南宁：广西科学技术出版社，2007.

［15］吕琳，曾振东．实用壮医诊疗技术操作规范［M］．南宁：广西科学技术出版社，2017.

［16］庞声航，王柏灿，莫滚．中国壮医内科学［M］．南宁：广西科学技术出版社，2004.

［17］庞宇舟，林辰．实用壮医学［M］．北京：北京大学出版社，2017.

［18］滕红丽，韦英才．民族医特色诊疗技术规范［M］．北京：中国医药科技出版社，2015.

［19］涂耀荣．浅谈针挑疗法［J］．中国民间疗法，1994（3）：25.

［20］韦英才．壮医经筋手法理论探讨及临床应用［J］．辽宁中医药大学学报，2012（6）：16-17.

［21］韦英才，梁子茂.壮医经筋学说理论浅探［J］.新中医，2017（12）：173-176.

［22］牙廷艺.壮医刮痧排毒疗法［M］.南宁：广西人民出版社，2009.

［23］牙廷艺.壮医针挑疗法［M］.南宁：广西人民出版社，2009.

［24］杨文进.壮医放血疗法的作用探讨［J］.中国民族医药杂志，1998，4（3）：33.

［25］曾振东，吕琳.壮医药物竹筒拔罐疗法技术操作规范与应用研究［M］.南宁：广西科学技术出版社，2007.

［26］钟鸣.壮医诊法技术规范［M］.南宁：广西科学技术出版社，2016.

［27］钟鸣.壮医技法技术规范［M］.南宁：广西科学技术出版社，2016.

［28］钟鸣.壮医病证诊疗规范［M］.南宁：广西科学技术出版社，2016.